In Clinical Practice

Taking a practical approach to clinical medicine, this series of smaller reference books is designed for the trainee physician, primary care physician, nurse practitioner and other general medical professionals to understand each topic covered. The coverage is comprehensive but concise and is designed to act as a primary reference tool for subjects across the field of medicine.

More information about this series at http://www.springer.com/series/13483

Rafael Díaz-Nieto
Editor

Procurement and Transplantation of Abdominal Organs in Clinical Practice

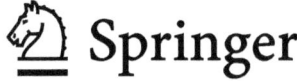 Springer

Editor
Rafael Díaz-Nieto
The Liver Unit
Aintree University Hospitals, NHS Foundation Trust
Liverpool
UK

ISSN 2199-6652   ISSN 2199-6660   (electronic)
In Clinical Practice
ISBN 978-3-030-21369-5   ISBN 978-3-030-21370-1   (eBook)
https://doi.org/10.1007/978-3-030-21370-1

This Springer imprint is published by the registered company Springer Nature Switzerland AG
The registered company address is: Gewerbestrasse 11, 6330 Cham, Switzerland

Acknowledgement

Authors would like to thank Professor Graeme Poston, Consultant Surgeon and Professor of Surgery at Liverpool University, for his kind collaboration in editing this manuscript.

Brief Introduction

This book was designed by the author based on the lack of general manuscripts that could summarize the main aspects of today's status of the procurement and transplantation of abdominal organs. This book has been created after some authors prepared the European Board accreditation in Transplantation Surgery; however, it cannot be considered the official material for its preparation. We would like to emphasize that this book does not describe in detail specific variations that can be found among the national protocols and for the daily practice of the transplant surgeons national and local protocols should prevail over this manuscript.

Contents

Chapter 1
Procurement of Abdominal Organs for Transplantation. Multiorgan Retrieval

Rafael Orti-Rodríguez and Rafael Díaz-Nieto

1.1 Relevant Concepts in Organ Donation and Types of Donors

1.1.1 Concept of Donation

General definition of donation is the act of giving something as a free contribution to someone (person or institution) who may need it. Therefore in the context of transplantation, a donor can be defined as a person who gives something (blood, tissues of body organs) so that it can be given to someone who needs it.

R. Orti-Rodríguez
Liver Transplant Unit Nuestra Señora de la Candelaria University Hospital, Tenerife, Spain

R. Díaz-Nieto (✉)
Hepatobiliary Surgery Unit, Aintree University Hospital, Liverpool, UK

Liver Transplant Unit Royal Free Hospital, London, UK
e-mail: rafael.diaz-nieto@nhs.net

© Springer Nature Switzerland AG 2019
R. Díaz-Nieto (ed.), *Procurement and Transplantation of Abdominal Organs in Clinical Practice*, In Clinical Practice,
https://doi.org/10.1007/978-3-030-21370-1_1

1.1.2   Types of Donors

– Living donor: alive person, and commonly healthy, who donates whole organs (kidneys), partial organs (liver) or tissues for the porpuses of transplantation and in a complete altruistic way.
– Deceased donor: person who donates organs and tissues after his/her death. Diagnosis of death can be made on the basis of neurological criteria (***Donation after Brain Death (DBD)***) or cardiocirculatory criteria (***Donation after Circulatory Death (DCD)***). Both are completely different entities in the context of organ procurement and require to be discussed separately.

1.1.3   Donation after Brain Death (DBD)

This is the most common type of donors nowadays in most of the occidental countries. It is important for the retrieval surgeon to understand the full scenario of a DBD from the diagnosis of death to the pathophysilolgy and perioperative management of these donors.

1.1.3.1   Definition of Brain Death

• *"Whole brain death"* is a clinical scenario that includes complete, irreversible, and definitive loss of brain, and brainstem functions.
• *"Brainstem death"* (generally used in the United Kingdom (UK)), and is based on irreversible cessation of all brainstem functions leading first to unconsciousness and respiratory arrest and, then to cardiac arrest.

1.1.3.2   Brain Death Aetiology

Aetiology of brain death can be any insult leading to irreversible damage of the brain/brainstem. The most common situations are:

- Cerebrovascular accident.
- Trauma.
- Hipoxia (secondary to any other origin).

1.1.3.3 Criteria and Diagnosis for Brain/Brainstem Death

Before establishing the diagnosis of brainstem death it is of crucial importance to exclude any potential causes, which can mimic brain death. This includes:

- Severe hypothermia (<33 °C).
- Hypoxemia.
- Shock.
- Metabolic encephalopaties such as liver failure, hypoglicemia, hypophosphoremia or hypothyroidism.
- Central Nervous System (CNS) depressant drugs such as alcohol, narcotics, muscular relaxants or hypnotic drugs.

Once we have excluded and/or corrected any of these situations we can consider our diagnosis based on the clinical scenario, detailed examination and some complementary tests.

Clinical diagnosis is based on a triad of coma, brain stem function cessation, and apnea.

A. Coma: lack of evidence of responsiveness. Eye opening or eye movement to noxious stimuli is absent. Noxious stimuli should not produce a motor response other than spinally mediated reflexes.
B. Lack of brainstem reflexes.

  – Bright light reflexes: Absence of pupillary response to a bright light is documented in both eyes. Usually the pupils are fixed in a midsize or dilated position (4–9 mm).
  – Absence of ocular movements using oculocephalic testing and oculovestibular reflex testing. Once the integrity of the cervical spine is ensured, the head is briskly rotated horizontally and vertically. There should be no movement of the eyes relative to head movement. The

oculovestibular reflex is tested by irrigating each ear with ice water (caloric testing) after the patency of the external auditory canal is confirmed. The head is elevated to 30 degrees. Each external auditory canal is irrigated (one ear at a time) with approximately 50 mL of ice water. Movement of the eyes should be absent during 1 min of observation. Both sides are tested, with an interval of several minutes.
- Absence of corneal reflex. Absent corneal reflex is demonstrated by touching the cornea with a piece of tissue paper, a cotton swab, or squirts of water. No eyelid movement should be seen.
- Absence of facial muscle movement to a noxious stimulus. Deep pressure on the condyles at the level of the temporomandibular joints and deep pressure at the supraorbital ridge should produce no grimacing or facial muscle movement.
- Absence of the pharyngeal and tracheal reflexes. The pharyngeal or gag reflex is tested after stimulation of the posterior pharynx with a tongue blade or suction device. The tracheal reflex is most reliably tested by examining the cough response to tracheal suctioning. The catheter should be inserted into the trachea and advanced to the level of the carina followed by 1 or 2 suctioning passes.

C. Apnea: Absence of a breathing drive. Absence of a breathing drive is tested with a CO_2 challenge. Documentation of an increase in $PaCO_2$ above normal levels is common practice.

*Apnea test:

- Adjust vasopressors to a systolic blood pressure >/=100 mmHg.
- Preoxygenate for at least 10 min with 100% oxygen to a PaO_2 >200 mmHg.
- Reduce ventilation frequency to 10 breaths per minute to eucapnia.

- Reduce positive end-expiratory pressure (PEEP) to 5 cm H2 O (oxygen desaturation with decreasing PEEP may suggest difficulty with apnea testing).
- If pulse oximetry oxygen saturation remains >95%, obtain a baseline blood gas (PaO2, PaCO2, pH, bicarbonate, base excess).
- **Disconnect the patient from the ventilator.**
- Preserve oxygenation (e.g., place an insufflation catheter through the endotracheal tube and close to the level of the carina and deliver 100% O2 at 6 L/min).
- Look closely for respiratory movements for 8–10 min. Respiration is defined as abdominal or chest excursions and may include a brief gasp.
- Abort if systolic blood pressure decreases to <90 mmHg.
- **Abort** if oxygen saturation measured by pulse oximetry is <85% for >30 s.
- Retry procedure with T-piece, CPAP 10 cm H2 O, and 100% O2 12 L/min.
- If no respiratory drive is observed, repeat blood gas (PaO2, PaCO2, pH, bicarbonate, base excess) after approximately 8 min.
- If respiratory movements are absent and arterial PCO2 is >/= 60 mmHg (or 20 mmHg increase in arterial PCO2 over a baseline normal arterial PCO2), the apnea test result is positive (i.e. supports the clinical diagnosis of brain death).
- If the test is inconclusive but the patient is hemodynamically stable during the procedure, it may be repeated for a longer period of time (10–15 min) after the patient is again adequately preoxygenated.

Complementary tests.
In clinical practice, electroencephalogram (EEG), cerebral angiography, nuclear scan, computered tomography with angiogram (CTA), and magnetic resonance (MRI/ MRA) are currently used as ancillary tests in adults. Most hospitals will have the logistics in place to perform and interpret an EEG, nuclear scan, or cerebral angiogram, and these 3 tests may be considered the preferred tests. Ancillary

tests can be used when uncertainty exists about the reliability of parts of the neurologic examination or when the apnea test cannot be performed. Some protocol use these tests to shorten the duration of the observation period. In adults, they are not needed for the clinical diagnosis of brain death and cannot replace a neurologic examination. There are also inherit disparities between tests and the potential for false-positives. Physicians may decide not to proceed with the declaration of brain death if clinical findings or complementary tests are unreliable.

1.1.3.4   Pathophysiology of Brain/Brainstem Death

Retrieval surgeons should understand the physiologic status of the donor prior to proceed with a multiorgan retrieval. Despite its complexity there is commonly a sequence of events that will impact in the metabolic situation. Some modificable factors may be managed in order to improve the haemodinamic situation of the donor and therefore the adequate perfusion and function of the organs to be retrieved.

- *Sequence*:
  - The increased intracranial pressure, secondary to oedema, may lead to an increased arterial blood pressure in order to ensure an adequate cerebral perfusion pressure.
  - The pontine ischemia can generate the so-called *Cushing reflex*. The Cushing's response is manifested with bradycardia and hypertension.
  - The ischemic damage will lead to an **autonomic storm** characterized with hypertension, tachycardia, and intense peripheral vasoconstriction. It is reported that the levels of catecholamines (adrenaline, noradrenaline, and dopamine) are greatly increased. This clinical scenario is often enriched with myocardial dysfunction secondary to increased oxygen consumption, arrhythmias, and increased myocardial contractility.

- After this hypertensive phase, hypotension may follow as a result of sympathetic outflow loss secondary to irreversible destruction of brainstem vasomotor nuclei.
- The autonomic storm causes an acute increase of left atrial pressure, increased pulmonary capillary pressure and pulmonary oedema.
- The later hypotension may be the result of **catecholamine depletion**, decreased cardiac output, myocardial dysfunction, intense peripheral vasodilatation, hypovolemia, electrolyte disorders, and endocrine changes.

Hypotension (mean arterial pressure (MAP) <50 mmHg or systolic arterial pressure (SAP) <60 mmHg) will represent ischemic damage of the future grafts with reduced graft survival.

- • *Modifiable factors*:
  - **Hypothermia** reduces heart rate and myocardial contractility, contributing to hypotension as well. Hypothermia may be related to loss of hypothalamic temperature regulation, large volumes of fluids administration, and opened cavities during surgery, and finally endocrine abnormalities. Hypothermia can also induce coagulopathy, hemolysis, and leftward shift of the oxy-hemoglobin dissociation curve.
  - **Electrolytes disturbances** (hypernatremia, hypokalemia, hypocalcemia, hypoMg) and acid-base disregulation.
  - Hypothalamic-pituitary abnormalities.
    - • Decreased thyroid function with myocardial consequences.
    - • **Diabetes insipidus** (polyuria, hypovolemia, hypotension, and hypovolemic hypernatremia) because of reduced Antidiuretic Hormone (ADH) production. Incidence of diabetes insipidus can reach up to 85% of brain dead donors.

- Reduced Adrenocorticotrope Hormone (ACTH) level, which is the primary mechanism for a **decreased cortisol** level.

*Hypotension, hypovolemia, bleeding, massive transfusions, brain death induced **inflammation**, and ischemia/reperfusion injury are important mechanisms that can cause hepatic dysfunction. The accumulation of leukocytes in the hepatic microcirculation may cause apoptosis of Kuppfer cells and induce depletion of glycogen stores.*

1.1.3.5   Management of the Brain-Death Donor

Donor management should be the responsability of the doctor in charge of the Intensive Care Unit (ICU) and/or emergency room, unless otherwise stated in the protocol of the local donor hospital. It can vary between different clinical situations but basic concepts are of the greates value at aiming to presever the best organs quality. General advices are:

A. Mechanical ventilation: protective lung ventilation is advisable especially when lung donation is considered. Low FiO_2, increased respiratory rate and target pressure <35 mmHg, tidal volumen 6–8 ml/kg/Bw, Peep between 5 and 10 mHg.
B. Rigorous pulmonary test monitoring arterial blood gases is important to prevent atelectasias, pneumonia and provide adequate ventilation (PaO_2 80–100 mmHg, $PaCO_2$ 35–45 mmHg, O_2 Sat >95% and pH 7.35–7.45). Keep the airway clean with intermittent nasopharyngeal suction.
C. Hemodynamic goals are to maintain the Mean Arterial Pressure (MAP) around 60–80 mmHg, systolic blood pressure over 90–100 mmHg, heart rate less than 100 bpm, and central venous pressure (CVP) 6–10 mmHg. Additionally, the ideal Pulmonary Capillary Wedge Pressure should be 10–15 mHg. For adequate hemodynamic management, 2 or 3 IV lines (including 1 central line) should be in place.

D. Volume control: The combination of crystalloids and colloids seems the most logical strategy. Crystalloids are not expensive, but can extravasate, leading to peripheral and interstitial oedema. The colloids are expensive, can deteriorate the coagulation system, and cause allergic reaction but their main advantage is less extravasation and better vascular bed filling. For lung and pancreas procurement colloids are preferred over crystalloids because of less incidence and severity of oedema. As described before, the infusion should vary to achieve a CVP of 6–10 mmHg.

E. After each 1.5 liters of crystalloids, Gelofusin or other colloids should be administered. If Hb <9.6 g/dl or Ht <20% packed cells, CMV (Cytomegalovirus) negative, should be given.

F. The use of vasopresors to maintain donor stability has recently been reported to improve organ viability, leading to an increased recipient survival rate. Noradrenaline produce splanic vasoconstriction with amelioration of pancreatic, hepatic and renal flows, therefore some authors suggest combination with dopamine to increase renal flow or switch to adrenaline. If the donor remains hipotensive despite adequate rehydratation or if blood pressure falls <80 mmHg, catecholamine should be given. Preferably use dopamine (≤10 μg/kg/Bw/min) or Norepinephrin <0.2 μg/Kg/Bw/min. A higher dose of cathecolamines can reduce renal and hepatic perfusion and therefore, whenever possible, higher doses of cathecolamines should be avoided.

G. Administration of glucose and insulin may improve glycogen storage and preoperative glucose blood level control post-brain death as well as maintain glucose blood level control. Monitoring of serun glucose every 4 h is advisable.

H. Electrolyte disturbances like hypernatremia, hypomagnesaemia, hypocalcaemia, hypokalemia and hypophosphatemia as a result of diabetes insipidus (caused by a déficit in the production of anti-diuretic hormone) may be responsable for severe hemodynamic instability. Therefore, the United Network for Organ Sharing (UNOS) reported that administration of "triple therapy" (triiodothyronine (T3) or thyroxine (T4) combined with steroids and vasopressin) showed a significant improvement in 1-month survival rate of transplanted organs compared to those donors not receiving triple therapy.

The advised treatment regimen is composed by a bolus dose of 4 μg T3 followed by a continuous infusion of 3 μg/h, ADH 1 U loading dose and an infusion of 1.5 U/h or desmopressin (DDAVP) 2 U/12 h, insulin as needed to maintain normoglycaemia, adrenaline 0–0.5 μg/h and intermittent hydrocortisone 5 μg/kg.

I. Diuresis should be maintained at 1–2 ml/kg/Bw/h. If diuresis does not increase despite adequate hydration, pharmacological preservation of renal function can be achieved by loop diuretics and mannitol. Both drugs are thought to decrease renal oxygen consumption by their effect on Na/K- pump. It is known that this pump in order to be fully functional consumes energy; so blocking the pump may reduce the energy consumption. Decreased renal oxygen consumption prevents the renal cortex becoming fragile in the course of ischemia. Mannitol may increase renal blood flow and also be a free radical scavenger.

J. Avoid hypothermia. The loss of central temperature regulation can cause hypothermia. Hypothermia may contribute to bradicardia, myocardial depression and induces coagulopathy. Warming mattress, blankets and warming up infuson fluids can be used to restore body temperatura to 35 °C–37 °C.

K. Brain death may be responsable for severe coagulation disturbances. These disturbances are not contraindication for liver transplantation. In case of evident bleeding this can be potentially reversible with the use of transfusions of fresh frozen plasma (FFP).

L. Strict aseptic conditions are mandatory to prevent infection and a special care should be taken to rule out sepsis.

Prophylactic antibiotherapy may be warranted avoiding nephrotoxic and hepatotoxic drugs. Preferably amoxycilline 15 mg(kg BW 4dd or Cefazoline 15 mg/kg BW 4dd.

1.1.4   Donation after Cardiac/Circulatory Death (DCD)

Initially called "*non heart beating donors*", this type of donation in increasing significantly in most of the occidental countries in the last few years. The most common retrieved organs are kidneys with a similar outcome as DBD in terms of graft survival and graft function after 5 years post transplantation. However the incidence of primary non-function (PNF) or delayed graft function (DGF) with DCD kidneys is higher than with DBD grafts. Outcomes of DCD in liver transplantatios are worse than DBD livers in terms of short and long-term outcomes. Very meticulous selection of donors is of vital importance to improve outcomes. Based on that, an initial Consensus Conference in Paris 2008, established some criteria to accept a DCD donor for liver transplant:

– Age <50 yo.
– ITU stay <5 days.
– WIT<30 min.
– CIT <8 h.
– No steatosis.

Nowadays all these criteria have been massively extended.

1.1.4.1   Definition and Diagnosis of DCD

Retrieval of organs for the purpose of transplantation from patients whose death is diagnosed and confirmed using cardio-respiratory criteria. Diagnosis of death is made by a doctor (intensivist/anaesthetist), independent to the transplant team, after 5 min of asystole, lack of central arterial pressure and lack of central reflexes.

We would like to enphasize the fact that the doctor making the diagnosis must be independent to the transplant team and that the retrieval/transplant team must never interact with the donor before the diagnosis of death.

1.1.4.2   Types of DCD

There are two principal types of DCD: *controlled and uncontrolled*. Uncontrolled DCD refers to organ retrieval after a cardiac arrest that is unexpected and from which the patient cannot be resuscitated. Therefore potential donors are brought into hospital dead or death is declared in hospital after unsuccessful resuscitation. In contrast, controlled donation ocurrs when planned withdrawal of life-sustaining treatments takes place on an intensive care unit, theatres or emergency department.

The clinical circumstances in which DCD can occur are described by the Maastricht classification (Consensus meeting held in Maastritcht in 1995 and modified in Madrid in 2011), Table 1.1:

1.1.4.3   New Concepts and Time of DCD

Recent expansion of DCD in most of occidental countries carries with a variation in the traditional retrieval process from a DBD. Times are now completely different and more complex that the standar cold and warm ischaemia times. The retrieval surgeon needs to be familiar to these terms and clearly understand their significance and relevance for the survival of the future grafts.

Times are actually different for DBD and controlled and uncontrolled DCDs. Nevertheless, all these times are variable and might be redefined with the used of normothermic perfusion machines.

"Concepts and times":
Controlled DCD (Fig. 1.1):

TABLE 1.1 Maastricht classification for DCD

Uncontrolled DCD	I	Death Occurring outside of hospital	To be a potential donor death has to be witnessed, the time that it occurred documented and resuscitation continued after death.
	II	Unsuccessful Resuscitation	**IIa**. Collapse occurs outside of hospital and death is confirmed on admission after continuous resuscitation manoeuvres.
			IIb. Collapse occurrs in hospital and resuscitation immediately started but unsuccessful.
Controlled DCD	III	Awaiting cardiac arrest	Death is inevitable but brain stem death criteria are not fulfilled. Treatment is withdrawn and death follows.
	IV	Cardiac arrest in a brain stem dead donor	Death has been diagnosed by brain stem criteria but patient suffers a cardiac arrest. This may be while awaiting the donor team or as an intentional arrangement (wishes of the next of kin).
	V	Unexpected cardiac arrest in a hospitalised patient	

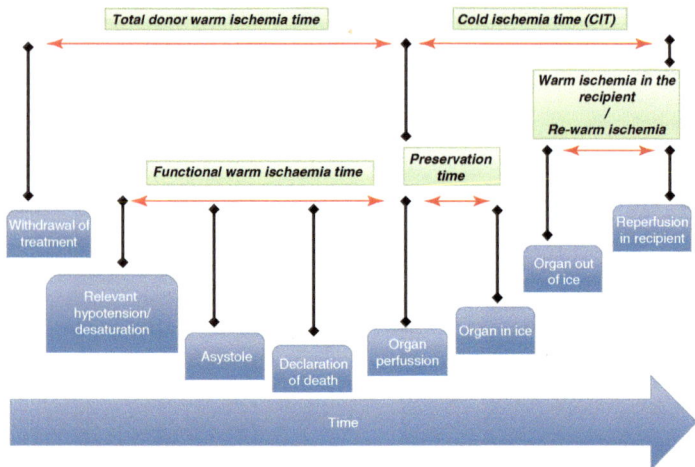

FIGURE 1.1 Diagram of the most relevant time and events for controlled DCD: Illustration of the normal vascular anatomy of the coeliac trunk and superior mesenteric artery with some of the most common anatomical variations

(a) **Withdrawal of treatment**: time for support cessation.
(b) **Time of relevant hypoperfusion**: time from when systolic BP (sustained at least 2 min) drops below 50 mmHg and Saturation below 70% (current recommendations: oxygen saturation below 70% is not used as an indicator of poor outcome or as a reason for non usage, but the retrieval team should keep record of when oxygen saturation falls below 70% in order to allow correlation with graft outcome.)
   In case of recuperation the time would be considered from first episode of these characteristics.
(c) **Asystole**: time of cardiac arrest. Where cardio-respiratory criteria apply, death can be confirmed following 5 min of continuous cardio-respiratory arrest providing there is no subsequent restoration of artificial cerebral circulation. Where possible, circulatory arrest should be identified by the absence of pulsatile flow on a correctly functioning arterial line, or by the use of echocardiography if the expertise is available; or failing that by continuous ECG monitoring. When treatment is withdrawn in Maastricht

type IV donors, death has already been declared and there is no need to verify death.

(d) **Total warm ischemia time**: time from treatment withdrawal to start of the preservation perfusion.

(e) **Functional warm ischemia time**: time from BP/Sat. drop to preservation.

(f) **Preservation time**: from start of the preservation manoeuvres to retrieval. Variable if perfusion, circulation machine (ECMO) used, otherwise should be minimal.

Uncontrolled DCD (Fig. 1.2):

(a) **Time of cardiorespiratory arrest (down time)**: time from arrest (witnessed) to start of cardiopulmonary resuscitation.

(b) **Time of resuscitation**: time from start of resuscitation to start of preservation manoeuvres (ECMO). This period can be divided in outside and inside-hospital.

(c) **Total warm ischemia time**: time from arrest to start of the preservation manoeuvres.

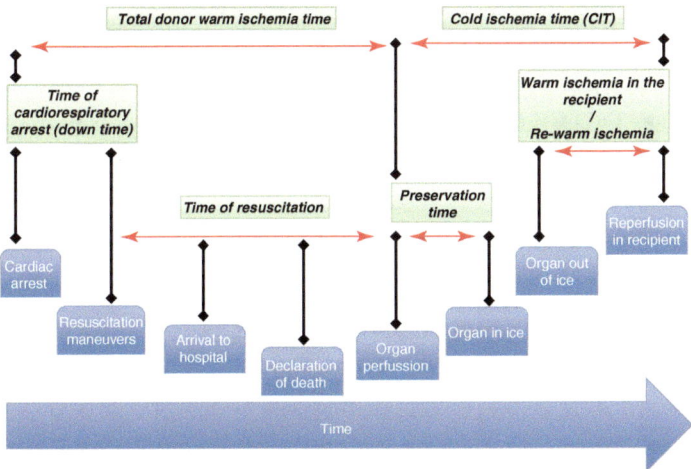

FIGURE 1.2 Diagram of the most relevant time and events for uncontrolled DCD: Illustration of how to perform an adequate arterial patch at the time of kidney retrieval

(d) **Preservation time:** from start of the preservation manoeuvres to retrieval.

– *Cold ischemia time* **(CIT)**: time from cold perfusion starts to implantation. Equal for any type of donor.

  * Some authors propose that the term CIT should not be used anymore due to the difficulties in measuring this time period (the time span between when the organ is effectively cooled down and when is it warmed up again, after removal from the transport box).

– *Warm ischemia in the recipient/Re-warm ischemia*: some authors support this concept as time from removal of the organ from the icebox to reperfusion.

DBD:
Concepts for DBD are equivalent and simplier since asystolia and start of perfusion occur at the same time. Therefore, ideally warm ischaemia time in the donor should be zero.
In general:

– **Total ischemic time:**

  • DBD: time between closing of the arterial clamp in the donor and start of the perfussion (generally called cross-clamp time) until the moment of releasing the arterial clamp in the recipient.

  • DCD: time between cardiac arrest in the donor until the moment of releasing the arterial clamp in the recipient.

– **Procurement time**: time between cross-clamp in the donor until placing the organ in the transport box (in case of cold storage) or connected to the perfusion machine.

– **Anastomosis time:** time from the extraction of the organ out of ice until arterial arterial.

All these times are important since organ tolerance to ischemia time is variable. As summary, Table 1.2 *shows approximate time of organs tolerance to ischaemia:*

TABLE 1.2 approximate ischaemia times tolerated by organ

	Warm ischaemia time	Cold ischaemia time
Kidney	45–60 min	24 h
Liver	30–45 min	8–12 h
Pancreas	45–60 min	18 h

1.2   Evaluation of Donor Suitability

1.2.1   Selection Criteria for Donation

Selection criteria for donors are based on an analysis of the risks related to the use of the specific cells/tissues. Indicators of these risks must be identified by physical examination, review of the medical and behavioural history, biological testing, post-mortem examination (for deceased donors) and any other appropriate investigation. We describe in this chapter general exclusion criteria for donors as well as organ-specific exclusion criteria. Again they are all general considerations that can vary between countries. Review of local policies is always advised.

1.2.1.1   Donor Exclusion Criteria

Unless justified on the basis of a documented risk assessment approved by the responsible person as defined in Article 17 of Directive 2004/23/EC, donors must be excluded from donation if any of the following criteria applies:

Deceased Donors

General Criteria for Exclusion

- **Cause of unknown death**, unless autopsy provides information on the cause of death after procurement and none

of the general criteria for exclusion set out in the present section apply. It is mandatory to obtain written consent from Coroner before proceeding with the retrieval.
- **History of a disease of unknown aetiology**.
- **Presence, or previous history, of malignant disease** (further discussion below), except for primary basal cell carcinoma, carcinoma in situ of the uterine cervix, and some primary tumours of the central nervous system that have to be evaluated according to scientific evidence. Donors with malignant diseases can be evaluated and considered for cornea donation, except for those with retinoblastoma, haematological neoplasm, and malignant tumours of the anterior segment of the eye.

- **Risk of transmission of diseases caused by prions**. This risk applies, for example, to:
  - (a) people diagnosed with Creutzfeldt–Jakob disease, or variant Creutzfeldt-Jacob disease, or having a family history of non-iatrogenic Creutzfeldt-Jakob disease;
  - (b) people with a history of rapid progressive dementia or degenerative neurological disease, including those of unknown origin;
  - (c) recipients of hormones derived from the human pituitary gland (such as growth hormones) and recipients of grafts of cornea, sclera and dura mater, and persons that have undergone undocumented neurosurgery (where dura mater may have been used).

- **Systemic infection which is not controlled at the time of donation**, including bacterial diseases, systemic viral, fungal or parasitic infections, or significant local infection in the tissues and cells to be donated. Donors with bacterial septicaemia may be evaluated and considered for eye donation but only where the corneas are to be stored by organ culture to allow detection of any bacterial contamination of the tissue (further discussion below).
- **History, clinical evidence, or laboratory evidence of HIV, acute or chronic hepatitis B (except in the case of persons with a proven immune status), hepatitis C and HTLV I/II,**

transmission risk or evidence of risk factors for these infections.

- **History of chronic, systemic autoimmune disease that could have a detrimental effect on the quality of the tissue to be retrieved**. This could includes colagenosis, massive arteriosclerosis and visceral repercussion from severe hypertension or diabetes. Most of the time is very difficult to have an organ assessment with lab tests and radiological investigations and a surgical assessment is necessary.
- **Evidence of any other risk factors for transmissible diseases** on the basis of a risk assessment, taking into consideration donor travel and exposure history and local infectious disease prevalence.
- **Presence on the donor's body of physical signs implying a risk of transmissible disease(s)**.
- **Ingestion of, or exposure to, a substance (such as cyanide, lead, mercury, gold) that may be transmitted to recipients in a dose that could endanger their health.**
- **Recent history of vaccination with a live attenuated virus where a risk of transmission is considered to exist.**
- **Transplantation with xenografts.**

Other Criteria for Exclusion

- **Age.** There is no clear limit of age for organ donation and depends on specific guidelines of each country. Donors older than 80 years old are being reporting more and more often.

Additional Exclusion Criteria for Deceased Child Donors

- Any children born from mothers with HIV infection or that meet any of the previous exclusion criteria must be excluded as donors until the risk of transmission of infection can be definitely ruled out.

  (a) Children aged less than 18 months born from mothers with HIV, hepatitis B, hepatitis C or HTLV infection, or at risk of such infection, and who have been breast-fed by their mothers during the previous 12 months, cannot be considered as donors regardless of the results of the analytical tests.

(b) Children of mothers with HIV, hepatitis B, hepatitis C or HTLV infection, or at risk of such infection, and who have <u>not</u> been breastfed by their mothers during the previous 12 months and for whom analytical tests, physical examinations, and reviews of medical records do not provide evidence of HIV, hepatitis B, hepatitis C or HTLV infection, can be accepted as donors.

Living Donors

The same exclusion criteria must be applied as for deceased donors in terms of risks for the recipient (trasmission of disesases). Nevertheless, additional exclusion criteria apply to avoid additional risks to the donor.

Special attention require pregnancy and breastfeeding. They are general exclusion criteria for living and deceased donation except for donation of umbilical cord blood cells and amniotic membrane and sibling donors of haematopoietic progenitors.

Living donation is very different depending on the organ to be retrieved therefore there are particularities that need to be described separately.

Possible Exlussion Criteria for Liver Living Donation

1. Age <18 yo (despite some oriental countries describe a minimum age of 16 yo) and <60 yo (variable between centres).
2. Diabetes.
3. History of thrombosis and/or embolism.
4. Haematological disorders.
5. Uncontrolable physiquiatric disorder.
6. Morbid obesity.
7. Coronary of peripheral vascular disease.
8. Previous liver disease (including alpha 1 antitrypsin).
9. Vascular of biliary abnormalities that may increase the likehood of failure.
10. Insufficient donor future liver remant or inadequate graft to body weight ratio.

Possible Exlussion Criteria for Kidney Living Donation

1. Age <18 yo.
2. Hypertension (BP >130/90 mmHg).
3. Diabetes.
4. History of thrombosis and/or embolism.
5. Haematological disorders including.
6. Psychatric contraindication.
7. Morbid obesity.
8. Coronary of peripheral vascular disease.
9. Urologic abnormalities.
10. Proteinuria.
11. Creatinine clearance <80 ml/min/1.73m^2.
12. Kidney stones (relative contraindication).

1.2.1.2   Organ-Specific Exclusion Criteria

Liver

- Cirrhosis.
- Portal vein thrombosis.
- Acute hepatitis (serum AST or ALT>1000 IU/L). Critical consideration of a potential derangement of the liver function tests is required as it can be justified by hipotensive episodes and it is potentialy reversible.
- Severe trauma.
- Severe enolism/steatohepatitis (following biopsy).
- HBV and HVC can be considered as relative contraindications (see below).

Kidney

- CKD (stage 3B or worse, eGFR<45).
- Long term dialysis (not acute relating to acute illness).
- Atrophic kidneys.
- Proteinuria >1 g/l.
- Haematuria of unknown origin.
- Staghorn calculi.
- Renal malignancy (see below)

Pancreas

- Insulin dependent diabetes (excluding ICU associated insulin requirement).
- Non-insulin dependent diabetes (Type 2).
- Any history of pancreatic malignancy.
- Donor Body Mass Index (BMI). There is no clear consensus about the limit of donor BMI. Even more, there are different limits wheter the pancreas is retrieved for islets only or to be used as a whole graft. It is demonstrated that there is a clear correlation between donor BMI and fatty infiltration of the pancreas.
- Donors Weight. The same problem happens when we talk about donor weight. There is no clear consensus about the lower limit of a donor weight. However in some countries it is accepted a pancreatic graft from a donor with less than 15 kg.
- Donor Age. There is no consensus and it is important to rely on national policies.
- Enolism/History of pancreatitis/Amylase-Lipase >2× normal limits. These are risk factors and markers of pancreatic damage but can be considered as relative contraindications.
- ITU stay longer than 7 days (for islets only).

Intestine

- Haemodinamic instability.
- Long cardiopulmonary arrest (consider recovery of hepatic and renal function as indicator of good flow recovery therefore bowel can be used).
- High doses of inotrops.
- Bigger size/weight than recipient (ideal 50–75% of the donor).
- CIT >8 h.
- ABO incompatibility.
- CMV positive.
- Age >55 yo.

1.2.2 Donor Transmissible Diseases

1.2.2.1 Tumours and Neoplasms

Generally speaking, diagnosis of neoplasm or lymphoproliferative disorder in the donor is contraindication for donation.

Exceptions

- **10 years disease-free survival.** In cases of adequate control during this follow-up period and in presence of proper investigations (imaging and or tumour markers) most of tumours can be considered cured after 10 yeras. Although controversial for some authors this exception is not applicable to some tumours (due to the higher risk of long term metastasis/recurrence) as:

  - Melanoma.
  - Breast cancer.
  - Soft tissue Sarcoma.

- **In-situ carcinomas.** Due to their low risk of metastasis but again excluding:

  - Melanoma.
  - Breast cancer.
  - Coriocarcinoma.
  - Lung cancer.

- **Non-melanoma skin cancer.** Any type of basocelular epitelioma or spinocellular carcinoma. Never melanoma as an exception even after 10 years disease-free survival or in-situ melanoma.

- **Renal Cell Carcinoma (RCC).** Donating a kidney with a RCC can be accepted if:

  - Resectable tumour.
  - Free Margins.
  - Tumour <4 cm.
  - No capsular involvement.
  - Fuhrman grade I-II (Table 1.3).

TABLE 1.3 Fuhrman classification for RCC

Fuhrman (nuclear) grade:

I	Small, round, uniform nuclei (10 microns), inconspicuous nucleoli, look like lymphocytes (very rare)
II	Slightly irregular nuclei, see nucleoli at 40× only, nuclear diameter 15 microns, open chromatin [40% of tumors]
III	See nucleoli at 10×, nuclei very irregular, diameter 20 microns, open chromatin [30–40% of tumors]
IV	Mitoses; bizarre, multilobated, pleomorphic cells plus grade 3 features, macronucleoli [15% of tumors]

- **Prostate cancer:** low risk transmission for Gleason score <6.

  *Gleason score system** is used to help evaluate the prognosis of men with prostate cancer using samples from a prostate biopsy. Pathologists sum the most often and the second most often histological patterns seen in the prostate biopsy. Patterns are classified with a number from 1 (cancerous propstate closely resembles normal prostate tissue) to 5 (the tissue does not have any or only a few recognizable glands) obtaining the final Gleason score (from 2 to 10)
- **Central Nervous System tumours.** Transmission risk is variable depending on the risk of extracranial dissemination and histology.

Few factors have been described as risk factors for transmission. Any of them increase the transmission from low risk to a high risk, being the transmission rate without risk factors of 7%; while of 36–43% in the presence of some of these factors factors.

Commonly accepted risk factors, described by Israel Penn International Transplant Registry are:

- Previous Surgery/Craniotomy (other than uncomplicated biopsy).
- Previous radiotherapy.
- Extra CNS mets

TABLE 1.4 WHO classification of CNS tumours

WHO Classification grade	
G I	Well differentiated (low grade)
G II	Moderately differentiated (intermediate grade)
G III	Poorly differentiated (high grade)
G IV	Undifferentiated (high grade)

– Ventricular derivation.
– Histological grade (WHO Classification grade III-IV) (Table 1.4).

Every case must be discussed individually but general consideration is that WHO grade I and II are not contraindication for donation and only some exceptions for grade III can be considered. Grade IV tumours are definitive contraindication for donation. Table 1.5 summarizes the most common situations.

Transmission risk can be classified in:

• No significan risk (frequency estimate 0%)
• Minimal risk (0–0.1%).
• Low risk (0.1–1%).
• Intermediate risk (1–10%).
• High risk (>10%).
• Unknown risk.

The use of intermediate and high risk donors is generally not recommended but an individual and specific evaluation of each case is required. Informed consent is mandatory from the recipient. In case of transmission of a neoplasia to the recipient it is mandatory to consider further treatment. It can consist on chemotherapy, explantation of the graft and retransplantation if needed.

1.2.2.2 Infections

As mentioned before the risk of transmiting a disease from the donor to the recipient is a contraindication for the donation.

TABLE 1.5 CNS tumours and donation

CNS tumours and donation	
Contraindication for donation	Glioblastoma multiforme
	Meduloblastoma
	Malignant ependimoma
	Pineoblastoma
	Malignant meningioma
	Sarcoma
	Cordoma
	Cerebral lymphoma
No contraindication for donation	Benign meningioma
	Pituitary adenoma
	Schwannoma
	Craniofaringioma
	Astrocitoma
	Hemangioblastoma
	Ganglioglioma
	Pineocitoma
	Oligodendroglioma
	Ependimoma
	Teratoma
Exceptions for WHO grade III tumours that can be considered for donation	Anaplastic meningioma
	Anaplastic astrocytoma
	Anaplastic oligodendroglioma
	Anaplastic oligoastrocitoma
	Anaplastic ependimoma

Infectious diseases are transferable to the recipient via the transplanted organ or tissue. However, due to the wide variety of infectious agents, the potential of treatment and the different intectious status of the recipient, there are many exceptions to this general contraindication.

General Contraindications for Donation

Donors with one of the following criteria should not be considered as potential donors unless especific considerations:

- Septicemia.
- Severe sepsis/septic shock (uni/multiorgan failure).
- Fungemia.

Particular Contraindications

- **HIV*:** It is a contraindication even for positive recipients. **Disease but not HIV infection alone (very controversial).*
- **HBV:** anti-HBs (surface) positive has low risk of transmission and it does not represent a contraindication. Anti-HBc (core) or HBV-Ag have high risk of transmission and can be only considered for positive recipients. Treatment with immunoglobulin (+/− lamivudine) would be indicated.
- **HCV:** It is not a contraindication in positive recipients. PCR is needed to assess viremia, which is a prognostic factor. Addtionaly a liver biopsy is suggested to assess the presence and degree of fibrosis.
- **HDV (Delta):** It is a potential coinfection with HBV and it represents a risk of primary fulminant hepatitis in the recipient.
- **HTLV I/II:** It is a contraindication in case of positive test, however this is not performed routinely. It carries a low risk of transmission.
- **EBV (*Epstein-Barr*):** It is not a contraindication but a risk factor for future lymphoproliferative disorders.
- **CMV:** No contraindication for liver, kidney or pancreas but clear contraindication for bowel transplant. It carries a high risk of primary infection in the recipient; therefore prophylaxis might be indicated (vanganciclovir).
- **WNV (Western Nile virus):** Contraindication. The risk of meningoencephalitis is significant.
- **Tuberculosis:** active infection is a contraindication while chronic/passed infection is contraindication only for lung transplant.
- **Meningitis from *Listeria Monocitogenes and M. Turberculosis:*** Contraindication.
- **Herpetic encephalitis:** Contraindication.
- **Disseminated hidatidosis:** Contraindication.
- ***Aspergillus spp.*:** Contraindication for lung transplant.
- ***Treponema Pallidum* (Sifilis):** No contraindication. Consider prophilaxis with Penicilin.
- ***Toxoplasma Gondii:*** Contraindication only for cardiac transplant.

- *Piercing and tattoos: they may represent an additional risk for transmittable infection. Considering the window period, if the tattoo/piercing was placed before the last 3 months they do not represent a contraindication. If there is a concern or a more recent act, serology may not be appropriate therefore PCR should be used. Investigations are also advised regarding the hygienic conditions of the place where the tattoo/piercing took place.*

1.2.3   Laboratory Tests Required for Donors

Based on the risk of any transmissible disease basic tests should be performed on the donor in order to identify active infectious diseases and or chronic infections potentially dangerous for the recipient. Once more, this book is a general view of the most common scenarios while there might be small modifications and peculiarities in every national protocol.

It is of the greates interest for the retrieval surgeon to know all these tests so they are checked before starting the harvesting of organs. A very important issue to consider regarding infection transmission is the concept of "***Window period***": time from some virus infection (HIV, HBC, HCV) to positive tests in serology. This time is variable but can reach up to 3 months. As alternative, HIV antigen or viremia (HCV) with PCR (polimerasa chain reaction) can be tested.

1.2.3.1   Biological Tests Required for Donors

- The following biological tests must be performed for all donors as a minimum requirement:
  - Anti-HIV-1,2
  - HBsAg and Anti HBc
  - Anti-HCV-Ab

Others:

- HTLV-I antibody testing must be performed for donors living, or having spent long periods, in areas of high-incidence.
- When anti-HBc is positive and HBsAg is negative, further investigations are necessary with a risk assessment to determine eligibility for clinical use.
- A validated testing algorithm must be applied to exclude the presence of active infection with Treponema pallidum. A non-reactive test, specific or non-specific, can allow tissues and cells to be released. When a non-specific test is performed, a reactive result will not prevent procurement or release if a specific Treponema confirmatory test is non-reactive. A donor whose specimen tests reactive on a Treponema-specific test will require a thorough risk assessment to determine eligibility for clinical use.
- In certain circumstances, additional testing may be required depending on the donor's history and the characteristics of the tissue or cells donated (e.g. RhD, HLA, malaria, CMV, toxoplasma, EBV, Trypanosoma cruzi).

1.2.3.2   General Requirements to Be Met for Determining Biological Markers

- The biological tests will be carried out on the donor's serum or plasma; they must not be performed on other fluids or secretions such as the aqueous or vitreous humour unless specifically justified clinically using a validated test for such a fluid.
- When potential donors have lost blood and have recently received donated blood, blood components, colloids or crystalloids, blood testing may not be valid due to haemodilution of the sample. An algorithm must be applied to assess the degree of haemodilution in the following circumstances:

(a) ante-mortem blood sampling: if blood, blood components and/or colloids were infused in the 48 h preceding blood sampling or if crystalloids were infused in the hour preceding blood sampling;

(b) post-mortem blood sampling: if blood, blood components and/or colloids were infused in the 48 h preceding death or if crystalloids were infused in the hour preceding death.

Tissue establishments may accept tissues and cells from donors with plasma dilution of more than 50% only if the testing procedures used are validated for such plasma or if a pre-transfusion sample is available.

- In the case of a deceased donor, blood samples must have been obtained just prior to death or, if not possible, the time of sampling must be as soon as possible after death and in any case within 24 h after death.
- In the case of living donors (except allogeneic bone marrow stem-cell and peripheral blood stem-cell donors, for practical reasons), or when tissues and cells of allogeneic living donors cannot be stored for long periods and repeat sampling is therefore not possible, blood samples must be obtained at the time of donation or, if not possible, within 7 days post donation (this is the 'donation sample').
- Where tissues and cells of allogeneic living donors can be stored for long periods, repeat sampling and testing is required after an interval of 180 days. In these circumstances of repeat testing, the donation sample can be taken up to 30 days prior to and 7 days post donation.
- If in a living donor the 'donation sample' is additionally tested by the nucleic acid amplification technique (NAT) for HIV, HBV and HCV, testing of a repeat blood sample is not required. Retesting is also not required if the processing includes an inactivation step that has been validated for the viruses concerned.
- In the case of neonatal donors, the biological tests may be carried out on the donor's mother to avoid medically unnecessary procedures upon the infant.

***Ambiguous or unconclusive virology result.** In case of doubt (i.e. the lab technician cannot say whether the result is positive or negative, a donor received several blood transfusions without the possibility to perform the test on a pre-transfusion blood sample) the organs of these donors should be matched and allocated assuming a positive virus result. Whenever possible a second test should be performed. If this test result is negative and the organ has not been allocated yet, a new match using the negative test result should be made. Then the organ should be allocated according to the new match result.

1.2.4 Extended Criteria Donor (ECD)

Once absolute and relatives contraindication have been excluded a donor can be considered suitable. Even at this stage we will face a wide variety of donors and there are many factors that will impact on the final outcome of the transplantation and the quality of the transplanted organ. The full transplant team (mainly the implanting team but also the retrieval team) needs to be aware of these entire donor's factors for proper allocation of the organs to the most suitable recipient.

Based con current multivariable analysys and large series of transplant many factors have been described. As summary and as general agreement from all these series, the most suitable donor would be:

A. White Caucasian.
B. Aged 5–40 yo.
C. DBD.
D. Deceased by trauma/accident.
E. Normal BMI.
F. No diabetic.
G. Whole graft to be transplanted (specification for liver transplantation).

Out of this ideal donor and taking into account different risk factors, there is a wide range of donors considered as *suboptimal* or *"extended criteria donors"*. To increase the pool of available organs, since 1987 when extended criteria donors were defined for the first time, world-wide transplantation units start using not only the most suitable donor previously exposed.

Grafts with risk factors have and increased risk of graft failure during the first posttransplantation month given the correlation between ischemic-reperfusion injury and PNF or IPF and an increased risk of graft loss given the correlation with biliary problems and chronic rejection.

An exponential calculation of the risk of graft failure after liver transplantation considering all these factors is known as **Donor Risk Index (DRI)**. UK and US follow different index but both consider "Donor-related factors" and "Transplant-related factors" (Table 1.6).

DRI comes after obteining some donor's characteristics with a prediction capacity of posttransplantation graft loss. It is a retrospective study of more than 20,000 liver trasnplantations between 1998 and 2002. Feng et al. did not include liver

TABLE 1.6 Donor risk index summary for liver transplantation

	US DRI		UK DRI	
	Reference value	RR of increased risk	Reference value	RR of increased risk
Donor related factor				
Age	<40	1.53 for 61–70 yo 1.65 for >70 yo	Any	1.05 increase per decade
Race	White	1.19 for African-American	White	2.17 for non-white

TABLE I.6 (continued)

	US DRI		UK DRI	
Size	Height	1.07 increase per 10 cm decrease in height	NA	
Cause of death	Trauma (DBD)	1.16 for CVA 1.2 for other DBD 1.51 for DCD	NA	
Type of graft	Whole liver	1.52 for partial/split	Whole liver	1.93 for reduce/ split
BMI	NA		Any	1.01 increase per unit increase
Transplant related factor				
CIT	Any	1.01 increase per hour increase	Any	1.02 increase per hour increase
Regional use	Local use	1.11 for regional use 1.28 for national use	NA	

US DRI United States Donor risk index, *UK DRI* United Kingdom donor risk index, *RR* relative risk, *yo* years old, *NA* not applicable, *DBD* donation after brain death, *DCD* donation after circulatory death, *BMI* body mass index, *CIT* cold ischaemia time transplantations in patients below 18 years old or combined transplant. It is a Cox regression model wich has as endpoint the time till graft failure. Over 28 different donor variables known at the moment of the organ offer, just 7 of them reached estatistical signifficance. It is a continuos measurement with a score between 0 and 3.0. With a DRI of 1.0 or less there is a 3-year graft survival of 81% and 60% for a DRI of more than 2.0.

1.2.4.1   Donor-Related Factors

- *Age*: it is known that an elderly liver has a lower weight and volumen as well as decreased blood flow than a young organ. However its functional reserve and regeneration capacity probably play a significant role in its final outcome. Between 1987 and 1992 there was an increased use of donors oldder than 50 years from 2% to 17%, and currently a big number of donors is over 60 years, increasing the age of a suitable donor from 50 to 80–85 with good final outcomes.
- *Steatosis*: the accumultion of fat in the liver is becoming more and more frequent given the global epidemic of overweight and obesity. If the current rates of obesity and diabetes continue for another two decades, the prevalence of Non-Alcoholic Fatty Liver Disease in the US is expected to increase in 50% in 2030. Around 20% of potential donors present moderate to severe liver steatosis. There are two different types of steatosis. Macrovesicular steatosis when the vesicles (where the excess lipid accumulates in) are large enough to distort the nucleus of the cell; otherwise the condition is known as microvesicular steatosis where the small intracytoplasmic vacuoles accumulate in the centre of the cell. Macrovesicular steatosis is commonly associated with alcohol intake, obesity and diabetes (which are at the same time donor-related factors included in DRI from Feng et al). Microvesicular steatosis is associated to mitocondrial damage caused by viral infections, metabolic disease or even sepsis.

- While microvesicula steatosis does not increase the risk of graft disfunction, organs with more than 30% of macrovesicula steatosis have a 25% risk of PNF.
- *Type of graft*: Split-liver transplantation (SLT) was introduced to increase the pool of organs. Originally the division was done in-situ to reduce CIT and to prevent blood loss after reperfusion. Although SLT decreases the drop-out rate in the waiting list, several variables in combination with this type of graft as age over 60 years, urgent indications, long CIT (>7 h) and retrasnplantation increase the risk of graft failure and poor patient survival.

There are no differences between DCD and DBD in terms of graft survival when WIT is less than 30 min and CIT less than 10 h. Non-controlled DCDs are associated to a higher rate of PNF, IPF and biliary complications than DBD. It is acceptted a maximun time of 130 min of WIT.

1.2.4.2 Transplant-Related Factors

- *Ischemia time*: the damage caused by ischemia is one of the more important factors involved in the graft dysfunction. The CIT is an independent factor for the ischemic-reperfusion injury and subsequently for PNF. A long CIT is a risk factor for intrahepatic biliary stenosis aswell.

Similar to the liver DRI, the **Kidney Donor Risk Index** (KDRI) is the equivalent for kidney donation and it is an estimate of the relative risk of post-transplant kidney graft failure based on some characteristics of the donor.

Table 1.7 summarizes main characteristics that are used to calculate the KDRI:

1.3 The Retrieval

The retrieval itself is not just a surgical operation to harvest organs and tissues. The full process starts with the donor's preoperative evaluation and apropriate documentation and

Donor characteristics (KDRI)
Age
Height
Weight
Ethnicity
History of hypertension
History of diabetes
Cause of death
Serum creatinine
HCV status
DCD

TABLE 1.7 Donor risk index summary for kidney transplantation (KDRI)

HCV hepatitis C virus, *DCD* donation after circulatory death

detailed collection of data followed by a meticulous coordination and logistic organization betweenn all the teams involved. This first step commonly developed by the donor hospital and the national transplant body may be different between countries. The surgical procedure is a complex operation very particular and uncomparable to any other intervention. Harvesting high quality organs is the main objetive of the intervention always preserving outstanding manners and respect for the donor's deceased body. Finally, it is also of vital importance the adequate management of the organs while they are preserved and transport until they are implanted in the recipient. From the start of the intervention, it is commonly the retrieval team (retrieval surgeon) the responsible of warranting that organs are retrieved and preserved in optimal conditions.

1.3.1   Preoperative Work-Up

Before the procurement of tissues and cells proceeds, an authorised person must confirm and record:

(a) Donor identification (first name, family name and date of birth).
(b) Donor's demogrphics: age, sex, place of birth, recent trips.
(c) Donor's medical records. All potential sources of information should be explore, from relatives to recent hospital and historic medical notes. Direct contact with the general practitioner is advised.
(d) Complete donor's body examination.
(e) Mandatory test results including blood group and pregnancy test (when applicable).
(f) Certification of death (brainstem death certificate in case of DBD). As mentioned before, this test must be done by two different doctors, independant from the retrieval team and at two different times.
(g) Coroner's approval (if applicable).
(h) Consent form completed and signned.
(i) Dates and times of every action.

All the records must be clear and readable, protected from unauthorised amendment and retained and readily retrieved in this condition throughout their specified retention period in compliance with data protection legislation. Donor records required for full traceability must be kept for a minimum of 30 years after clinical use, or the expiry date, in an appropriate archive acceptable to the competent authority. In the case of living donors, the health professional responsible for obtaining the health history must ensure that the donor has understood the information provided and had an opportunity to ask questions and been provided with satisfactory responses.

1.3.2   Organ Procurement. The Surgical Technique

Despite some similarities, DBD and DCD have very different approaches and required different logistic preparation. A standar DBD can initially be considered as a normal surgical operation with a patient requiring adequate management from the anaesthetic point of view as for any other patient.

Therefore all the process of transferring the patient into theatre and starting the operation follows the same principle of an elective operation.

In contrast, DCD is completely different. Uncontrolled DCD may arrive to theatre already supported by a perfusion machine or extracorporeal membrane oxigenator machine (ECMO) or with the donor receiving constant cardiorespiratory resucitation manouvres. Controlled DCD will be transfer to theatre in asystoly therefore superurgent cannulation is essential. Because of this and in order to minimise warm ischaemia time, treatment withdrawal for DCDs is best done near to the operating theatre whenever is possible and retrieval teams must be present and scrubbed in theatre at the point of treatment withdrawal.

It is exclusive of controlled DCD the waiting time from withdrawal of treatment to asystoly and hence the starting of the operation. Regular monitoring of the donor's haemodinamics is essential to stablish the starting time of the functional warm ischaemia time. Maximum waiting time can be different between countries, being the agreed protocol in UK of 1 h waiting time to decline the use of the pancreas and the liver and three to four ours to stand down the kidneys. This is controversial specially in cases of complete haemodinamic stability of the donor for the full 4 h, however the suspected catecolamine storm and splanic compensation may hide a situation were abdominal organs are being poorly perfussed while vital constants are normal. National protocols should be followed in any case.

Observation of this, so called "agonal phase", has promote systems aiming at predicting the chances of the donor to achieve asystole. Wisconsin Criteria is shown in Table 1.8 as example.

1.3.2.1   Surgical Technique for DCD

Once death is confirmed, quick transfer to the operating table is essential (lights, table height, preservation solutions and cannulas must be set up). However, donor's identification

TABLE 1.8 Wisconsin Criteria considered as predictive factors (variable punctuation to each variable) Probability of progression to asystole after treatment withdrawal (type III only)

Age	
0–30	1
31–50	2
>50	3
Respiratory Rate after 10 min	
>12	1
<12	3
Abscence of respiratory movements	9
VT	
>200 ml	1
<200 ml	3
Negative Inspiratory Pressure	
>20 mHg	1
<20 mmHg	3
Inotropes	
No Inotropes	1
One	2
More than One	3
BMI	
<25	1
25–29	2
>29	3
Sat O2 after 10 min	
>90%	1

(continued)

TABLE 1.8 (continued)

80–89%	2
<79%	3
Orotracheal tube	3
Tracheostomy	1

Range from 8% possibility of death after 60 min. For 10 points to 98% for 23 points.

and verbal or written confirmation of death must be made prior to proceed.

Main steps are:

(a) Chest and abdomen are rapidly prepped and draped.
(b) Midline incision from supraesternal notch to the symphysis pubis. Quick laparotomy (no need for diathermy) and self-retaining retractor to keep the abdomen open.
(c) Sharp dissection of the right or left iliac artery to warranty perfusion of any renal polar arteries arising from the iliac arteries.

∗Minding the right ureter to avoid cutting it too short and to avoid any damage of iliac artery (prejudicing its use for reconstructing the arterial supply to the pancres), the right iliac artery should be cannulated as close to the aortic bifurcation as possible.

(d) Cannulation: insertion of a flushed ("air-free") cannula into the artery and tie distally and proximally.
(e) Venting/Perfusion: as soon as the cannula is inserted, the preservation solution can be perfused but draining the outflow of the organs it is recommended simultaneously to prevent congestion of the organs. Generally, another cannula/drain is inserted into the distal cava vein to keep the surgical field as dry as possible. Alternatively, venting can be done in the chest by transecting the supra-hepatic cava/right atrium. Blood should not accumulate in the chest as it may reduce the cooling of the organs.

If the donor is Maastricht type 4, the donor can be heparinised immediately before treatment withdrawal. This is not allowed for type 1,2 or 3 DCD donors and therefore the first two litres of preservation solution should be loaded with the appropriate dose of heparin (3–5 mg/kg or 500 U/kg). If both portal vein and aortic perfusion is to be undertaken, the first portal bag must also contain heparin.

(f) Surface cooling with iced-solution (mind frozen lesions). Ice around the liver, between the bowel loops, in the lesser sac and behind each kidney.

(g) Quick thoracotomy with Gigli or automated sternal saw for supracoeliac aorta clamping. Alternative clamp can be applied in the intraabdominal supracoeliac aorta (cases of difficult thoracotomy due to previous thoracic surgery) but exploratory thoracotomy is always suggested to assess the lungs. After aortic clamping, the perfusion fluid pressure can be increased to 200 mmHg.

(h) Additional venting from the right atrium.

(i) Surface cooling with saline ice slush in the right hemithorax on the dome of diaphragm above the liver.

(j) Liver retrieval: portal perfusion is paramount through Portal Vein, SMV or IMV. When concomitant pancreatic retrieval portal perfusion has to be made through PV approximately 1 cm from the edge of the duodenum.

(k) The common bile duct and the gallbladder is then divided and flushed with cold saline.

Once the organs are removed or during the cold flushing of the organs, it is time for a meticulous exploration of both cavities to assess any malignancy. The kidneys should be assessed by removal of the perinephric fat before cold storage.

**Particular of type II DCDs with lung donation is the insertion of chest drains for cold perfusion (2 for infusion and 2 for drainage), aiming an oesophageal temperature of 20 °C.*

¡¡!!*It is very important to assess adequate perfusion of all organs, otherwise recannulaton may be needed.*¡¡!!

1.3.2.2   Surgical Technique for DBD

As mentioned before, donor is transfer to the operation room under anaesthetic supervision like any other operation. Donor's identification is mandatory. There is an initial phase (warm phase) of disecction and preaparation of the organ for harvesting after perfusion (cold phase).

Warm phase steps:

(a) Midline laparotomy +/− thoracotomy +/− transverse (cross) laparotomy. Thoracotomy is suggested not only for exposure but also for lung assessment.

Tricks: divide round and falciform ligaments close to the abdominal Wall and the diaphragm up to hepatic veins as soon as laparotomy is done and before thoracotomy to avoid any damage of the liver.

Before the thoracotomy protect the liver with a large swab to avoid any damage (remember asking to anesthesist to deflate both lungs). After thoracic retractor is placed, use sterile wax and/or electrocautery to obtain adequate hemostasis and just before Finochietto retractor is opened, divide perycardium ("L" incision), both pleuras and cut anterior side of the diaphragm to avoid any bleeding or tears.

Additional advantage of thoracotomy: if retrograde cannulation is not feasible (massive arteriosclerosis, previous aortic surgery, aneurism…) the anterograde cannulation from the thoracic aorta is required.

(b) Full cavities exploration looking for tumors (malignancy), infection and/or injuries.
(c) Liver inspection. Examine the liver for its quality (steatossis, fibrosis, cirrhosis, edema), injury (tear, haematoma), tumor (benign, malignant) or infection (cholecystitis, cholangitis). Examine liver arterial blood supply in hepato-gastric and hepato-duodenal ligaments.
(d) Pancreas inspection (through hepatogastric ligament, gastrocolic ligament, detaching greater omentum from the transverse colon or using kocher manouvre just to

assess the head). Remember use the "no touch technique" looking for edema, tumors, fibrosis, injury hematoma and infection.

(e) Cattell-Braasch manoeuvre. Up to the dissection of the proximal 2 cm of the SMA in order to identify any aberrant hepatic anatomy. Keep in mind left renal vein, which usually crosses over the Aorta, and possible right accesory renal arteries that can cross the Vena cava.

Isolation with ties of the aorta distally to the renal arteries is suggested at this step so the cannulation can be performed quickly in case of donor instability. In order to avoid any damage to a possible aberrant renal artery, cannulation is recommended via right iliac artery close to the aortic bifurcation keeping always in mind the right urether. If this is the case, another tie has to be put around the left iliac artery to avoid perfusion solution loss going into the left lower limb.

It is useful to isolate IMA too. A prepared tie could avoid the useless reperfusion of the bowel if there is no intestinal retrieval.

(f) Dissection of the supracoeliac aorta for *crossclamping*. Access to this can be done through the chest or through the abdomen keeping in mind a possible damage of the oesophagus that should be recognised and retracted to the left. To visualize the abdominal aorta under the diaphragm divide the crura muscles of diaphragm from the hiatus to the celiac trunk. To get around the aorta is necessary to free it from all fibrous tissue around it.

(g) Full gastrolisis and division of gastro-colic ligament to expose and assess the pancreas. Short gastric vessels are divided close to the stomach and the tail of the pancreas is mobilised. Pull down the transverse colon and the greater omentum to achieve the optimal visualization of the mesenteric vessels and the transverse mesocolon.

(h) Mobilisation of right and left hepatic lobes. Isolation of SHVC or SHVeins is not recommended to avoid any damage.

(i) If pancreas is going to be retrieved it is helpful for the cold phase to put a nylon tape where a stapler will be used (pylorus, 1st jejunal loop and root of mesentery. A swap behind the spleen is useful to avoid any tear and easily lift it during the cold phase, using it as a handle to lift the pancreas from left to right.

(j) Hepatoduodenal ligament dissection.

  (i) Identification of aberrant anatomy (RAHA/LAHA). Always be very careful and look for the RAHA (location: right side of the portal vein, behind the common bile duct or common aberrant hepatic artery).

  (ii) Dissection, division and flush of the bile duct (1–2 cm above the pancreas). Can be done through the gallbladder although in some countries is avoided due to opening up the GB can lead to contamination.

  (iii) Dissection and isolation of the GDA (division only during the cold phase 5–10 mm from its origin in order to avoid CHA strictures). A previous identification and freedom of 1.5 cm of the common hepatic artery can be useful. Rubber slings are recommended as a mark for vessels instead of surgical ties to avoid any damage (vascular dissection).

  (iv) Dissection and isolation of the SA if DPA not arising from CHA (division only during the cold phase 5–10 mm form its origin in order to avoid CHA strictures).

  (v) Dissection of the PV in cases of pancreas retrieval (2–3 cm above the pancreas). In this case a tie is preferred instead of rubber slings giving the fact that we will use it to fix portal cannula.

    *All this dissection can be omitted in cases of in-block retrieval of the liver and pancreas for posterior division during the bench work. The bile duct can be flushed via the gallbladder.

    *Additionally, the portal vein can be cannulated either via SMV or IMV for combined perfusion. In cases with pancreas procurement, this cannulation *would compromise the pancreas outflow with the consequence congestion of the organ, hence, the PV can be cut (2 cm above the pancreas) during the cold phase and the portal cannula inserted for perfusion. To cannulate PV through SMV holding transverse colon up and dissecting in the right side of DJ flexure.*

(k) Heparinization (3–5 mg/kg or 300–500 U/kg).
(l) Ties should only be knotted and the common Iliac artery or Aortic cannula inserted 3 min after administration of heparin.
(m) Cannulation.
(n) **Crossclamp + perfusion + venting + surface cooling.**

As per protocol: perfusion with UW (75–100 ml/kg) or HTK (150–300 ml/kg) under pressure (300 mmHg) to warranty physiological aortic pressure (70–80 mmHg) and proper HA flow and organ perfusion.
Cold phase steps:

(a) Liver harvesting: Cut the inferior vena cava (IVC) just above the renal veins. It is useful to cut the patch from inferior vena cava with the left renal vein and reflect it. Through that cut, localize the ostium of the right renal vein to make sure you cut the IVC 1–1.5 cm obove the ostium of the right renal vein. Cut the diaphragm (left side, right anterior, lateral and posterior) staying away from the liver ligaments to avoid liver tearings or injuries and retracting the oesaphagus to the left. Divide the hepatogastric ligament should be divided close to the stomach wall starting from the pylorus to preserve left aberrant hepatic artery. Divide the gastroduodenal artery (GDA) (0.5 cm above the pancreas head), PV and SA (0.5 cm from the celiac trunk) marking the pancreas side of GDA and SA with the Prolene 5/0 suture. Putt he forefinger in the IVC to lift the liver and use it as a reference during dissection. Retroperitoneal dissection via the adrenal gland plane on the right side and the left side of the Aorta using as landmark the reference in SMA to avoid any damage of renal arteries. Aortic patch of the

Coelica trunk. Liver out. Procured the liver and place the liver in a sterile container filled with 4 °C preservation solution (no ringer or NaCl). The liver has to be flushed with minimum 500 ml of cold preservation solution. Inform recipient center of this as well as the quality of the result.

(b) Pancreas harvesting: Consider deinfection with betadine via NG tube. Divide with stapler the duodenum at the pylorus and Treitz ligament. Divisie mesenteric vessels and transvese mesocolon 3–5 cm centimetres distally from the inferior border of the pancreas/uncinate process using gastrointestinal or vascular stapling device or ligation. If GDA, PV and SA are already divided, then create an aortic patch around the ostium of the SMA. Proceed to a retroperitoneal dissection by cutting the spleen ligaments and freeing the pancreas from retroperitoneal attachments up to the left side of the aorta using the spleen as a "handle". Mind left renal arteries. Place the procured pancreas in a sterile container filled with ice and cold sterile 0.9%NaCl or Ringer's lactate or preservation solution.

Anatomical difficulties:
Anatomical variations (Fig. 1.3):
Warning and remember:

- 42% has the normal arterial blood supply: the common with proper hepatic artery with no additional arterial branches;
- 30% has the left aberrant hepatic artery coming from the left gastric artery and the normal liver arterial blood supply;
- 20% has the right aberrant hepatic artery coming from the superior mesenteric artery (SMA) and the normal liver arterial blood supply;
- 8% has both right and left aberrant hepatic arteries and the normal liver arterial blood supply;
- 3% of the population has a common aberrant hepatic artery coming from the SMA and no coeliac trunk and no common hepatic artery.

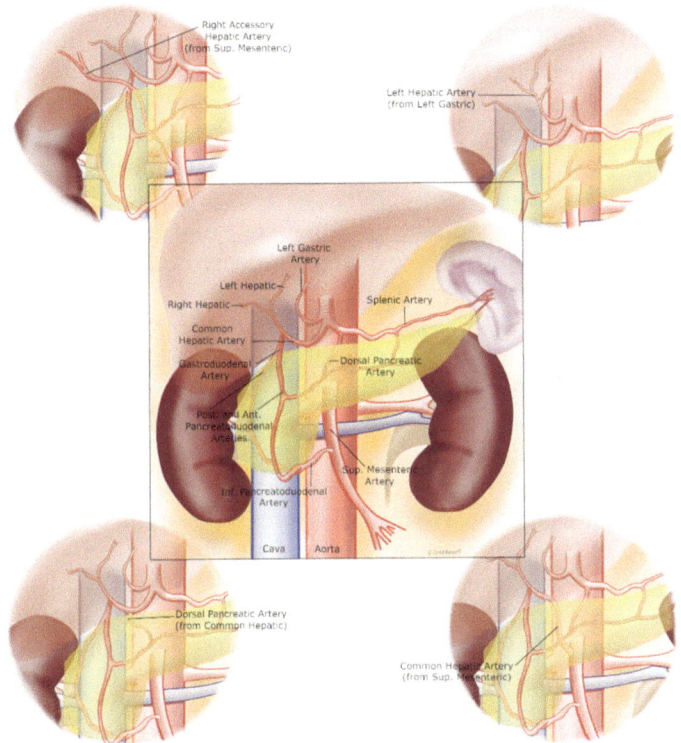

FIGURE 1.3 Anatomical variations

- **In the presence of an aberrant right hepatic artery with a complete extra-pancreatic course,** we can decide to dissect this artery close to its origin with 1 cm cuff or patch from the SMA.
- **In case of an intra-pancreatic right hepatic artery**, its division should only be done after consultation between pancreas and liver teams. If this artery is transected proximal to the pancreatic head, the liver surgeon must have the possibility to implant the right aberrant hepatic artery into the ostium of either gastroduodenal or splenic artery.
- **In case of the dorsal pancreatic artery is arising from the common hepatic artery or from the celiac trunk (or even**

from the GDA or arteries further away) the procurement surgeon has to communicate with the liver and the pancreas receiving center(s). In these two cases of anatomical abnormality the common hepatic artery has to be cut 3–5 mm from the celiac trunk and the celiac trunk and the SMA has to be given to the pancreas with the aorta patch.

• **In some cases (small children as donors and recipients, difficult adult recipient, no adequate "tool- kit" for organ reconstruction)** the pancreas procurement as a whole organ should be avoided.

(c) Kidneys harvesting: left vein is divided as above (does not need a patch of vein) followed by the division of the aorta (arterial abdnormalities are common therefore keep the full patch of aorta (Fig. 1.4) and assess for a possible retroaortic left renal vein). Mobilize then from midline to lateral and down to the pelvis preserving as much periureteric tissue as possible. The cava will go with the right kidney and can be used in case of a very small right vein. Warning! Be aware of the possible presence of a Right Aberrant Renal Artery arising from the common iliac artery and which could also course anterior to the vena cava. Be aware of it when freeing the Inferior Vena Cava.

(d) Bowel harvesting: in case of multivisceral transplantation we may need to retrieve in-block liver+pancreas+duodenum+bowel, pancreas+bowel or bowel independently. In this last scenario it is mandatory to preserve inferior branches from SMA and SMV to the pancreas (DPA can rise from SMA). First jejunal branches can be sacrificed.

(e) Iliac vessels Tool-Kit: It is necessary to deliver the common iliacal artery and vein with the bifurcation of the internal iliacal artery and vein with the pancreas. It is necessary to deliver the second set of common iliac artery and vein with the bifurcation of the internal iliacal artery and vein with the liver. It is extremely important to retrieve good quality vessels, as they may be required in case of complex vascular anastomosis.

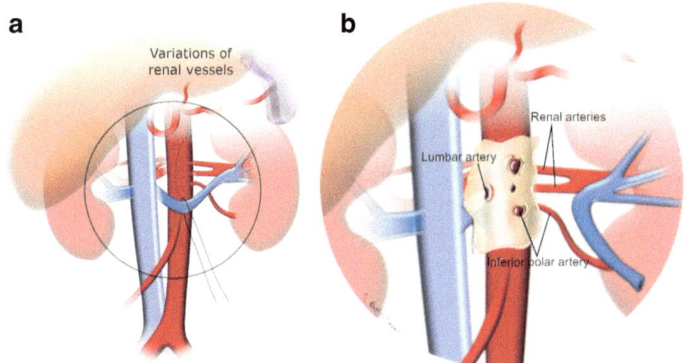

FIGURE 1.4 Aortic patch

Closure.

- Special consideration requires the closure. Majority of teams will choose to close only the skin but there is no clear indication against other layers'closure. What is of extreme relevance is the consideration and respectful management of the deceased body that might come back to the familiy to be burried. Irrespective the type of closure choosen, it has to be hermetic so residual fluid does not leak through the wound. Attention needs to be paid to cosmetic especially in case of any special request from the family.

Back table (organs always placed in bowls with ice saline slush):

(a) Remove periphrenic fat along the lateral border of the kidney.
(b) Assessment of perfusion and abnormalities.
(c) Complement perfusion if required.

1.3.3   Organ Assessment

Proper assessment of all the organs is mandatory. Not only those organ that are ment to be retrieved but also all the remaining organ and visceras in the abdominal and thoracic cavities. This assessment will happen in two occasions: at the time of laparotomy and once they have been removed from the body.

For DBD is recommended to make a meticulous exploration of the cavities as soon as entering into them while in cases of DCD priority is given to cannulation and only after the perfusion is running, there is adequate venting and surface cooling we can take some time to formally assess organs and visceras.

Aim of this exploration is seeking for:

  (i) Evidence of tumour: cancel the donation.
 (ii) Suspicious of tumour (including endometriosis): biopsy.
(iii) Inflammation (diverticulitis, appendicitis): proceed.
(iv) Other inflammation or free fluid: cultures/biopsy.

- **_Special situations: action to be taken._**

Evidence of tumour or any major alteration uncompatible with transplantation (cirrhosis, pancreatitis…) would be contraindication to proceed with the retrieval. However, it is very common to find small abnormalities that make the differencial diagnosis between malignant and benign diseases extremely difficult for the retrieval surgeon. Most of the transplant programs include access to histopathology for those cases that require confirmation and fluent communication with the implant team is essential in cases of doubts.

Some of the most typical situations for every organ are summarized.

- Liver assessment. Key features from the liver that need attention are colour, shape, size and edges. We can find relatively often some of these situations:

  1. Discoloured spots below the capsule.
  2. Capsule tear, haematoma or liver rupture: discuss with the implantation centre. May require further investigations regarding the extension of the damage.
  3. Enlarged, swollen liver with blunt edges: these moght be signs of a diseased liver but the need to be reassessed

after perfusion because it can be also related to *congestion after cardiac death or hypernatremia*

4. Fibrotic liver
5. Steatotic liver with blunt edges: needs discussion with the implant team and biopsy
6. Cirrhotic: it is an exclusion criteria
7. Enlarged nodes at the liver hilum
8. Palpable/Visible tumour: they need to be biopsied.

– Pancreas assessment. Very important characteristicts are size, fatty infiltration, softness, inflammatory changes and nodularity. Being typical scenarios:

   1. Small haematoma: discuss with the implantation team to decide the extension of the damage.
   2. Small, shrunken, hard pancreas: fibrotic pancreas. Probably unsuitable for transplantation.
   3. Slightly swollen pancreas: reevaluate after perfusion. Possible swelling due to hypernatremia or intracerebral oedema. Potentially correctable after perfusion.
   4. Swollen, fibrosed, inflamed: reject. Pancreatitis is contraindication.
   5. Irregular hard tumour: the pancreas will be rejected but it needs to be biopsied in case there are other organs retrieved that may need to be rejected.

– Kidney assessment: the procuring surgeon has the responsability to perform a thorough inspection of the kidneys by removing all the perirenal adipose tissue. Remind to preserv the fatty tissue around the renal hilus and avoid dissection near the lower pole in order to reduce risk of damaging the ureter vasculature.

   1. Quality of perfussion: patchy perfusion may represent a missed polar artery.
   2. Tumours/Cysts: biopsy should be taken tangentially and never perpendicular to the long axis due to the risk of pelvis damage.
   3. Staghorn calculi.
   4. Ureter length.

1.3.4   Packing (Cold Storage)

Once organs have been retrieved and reviewed, adequate packing is mandatory to warraty a safe transfer to the recipient hospital. Again some differences might be found among different countries but as general advises we can consider the following:

Each organ should be stored in three separate bags:

- The first bag is filled with 4 °C preservation solution.
- The first bag is put into the second bag which is filled with cooled saline or Ringer's lactate solution.
- The second bag is put into the third bag. It is recommended to keep the third bag dry.

All bags are de-aired and well tied. The organ is put into a transport box and well covered with non-sterile melting ice. Ice should never been in direct contact with the organs as frozen lesions have been described related to this.

Another requirement that is routine practice and we just briefly mention is that all organs should be transfer with one piece of spleen, good quality lymph nodes (para-aortic, small bowel or mesentery located) and blood specimen. The spleen and lymph nodes are to be put into tubes containing saline or Ringer's lactate solution which tubes are to be put into a labeled small box. Another piece of spleen is used for tissue typing and cross matching. This piece of spleen is stored in the same way as described above. Blood samples, lymph nodes and/or spleen for each abdominal organ should be properly and identically identified.

Labelling of the procured tissues/cells

At the time of procurement, every package containing tissues and cells must be labelled. The primary tissue/cell container must indicate the donation identification or code and the type of tissues and cells. Where the size of the package permits, the following information must also be provided:

(a) date (and time where possible) of donation;
(b) hazard warnings;

(c) nature of any additives (if used);
(d) in the case of directed donations, the label must identify the intended recipient.

If any of the information under points (a) to (d) above cannot be included on the primary package label, it must be provided on a separate sheet accompanying the primary package.

Labelling of the shipping container

When tissues/cells are shipped by an intermediary, every shipping container must be labelled at least with:

(a) TISSUES AND CELLS and HANDLE WITH CARE;
(b) the identification of the establishment from which the package is being transported (address and phone number) and a contact person in the event of problems;
(c) the identification of the tissue establishment of destination (address and phone number) and the person to be contacted to take delivery of the container;
(d) the date and time of the start of transportation;
(e) specifications concerning conditions of transport relevant to the quality and safety of the tissues and cells;
(f) in the case of all cellular products, the following indication: DO NOT IRRADIATE;
(g) when a product is known to be positive for a relevant infectious disease, marker the following indication: BIOLOGICAL HAZARD;
(h) in the case of autologous donors, the following indication: 'FOR AUTOLOGOUS USE ONLY';
(i) specifications concerning storage conditions (such as DO NOT FREEZE).

1.3.5   Donor Management and Organ Preservation

As result of hypoxia there is a reduction in the intracellular ATP (adenosin triphosphato) and therefore failure in the Calcium channels and Na-K ATPase pump. Thereafter there is intracellular accumulation of Ca, Na and water with hidropic degeneration and death of the cell.

In order to ameliorate this effect there are several preservation techniques and solutions that aim to:

(a) Preserve adequate pH.
(b) Avoid intracellular oedema.
(c) Provide metabolic support.
(d) Avoid free radicals (*Reactive Oxygen species*) damage.

Types of graft injury:

- *Pre-preservation injury*: injury present prior to preservation perfusion. Can be related to donor condition (liver esteatosis), heamodinamic situation of the donor or injuy during the harvesting.
- *Preservation injury.* Injury produced during the harvesting procees.
- *Cold preservation injury.* Despite hypothermia and adequate perfusion, the organ will suffer the effects of hypoxia consisting on cellular swelling, alteration of the cytoskeleton and extracellular matrix and final endothelial detachment into the sinusal lumen with consequent poor perfusion.
- *Rewarming injury*: injury related to the enzyme reactivation and metabolic rate. It is time-related therefore rewarming should be always less than 60 min.
- *Reperfusion injury*: complex mechanism involving reactive oxygen species, extracellular free iron (Fenton Reaction), cytokines from Kupffer cells activation and Neutophil activation (TNF-a and IL-1), proteases activity (Calpain and caspases) and nitric oxide.

Techniques to ameliorate the damage:

(a) **Hypothermia**: reduce metabolic rate. 1–4 °C reduce metabolic activity to 3–5% of normal metabolism.

In situ (intraluminal) flush with cold solutions reduce temperature <10 °C 3–5 min vs 20 min for surface cooling. Unfortunatelly 4 °C are only achieved once the organ in storaged convered in ice.

(b) **Preservation solutions**: provide basic substances for the cells (Table 1.9).

TABLE 1.9 summary and main characteristics of the most commonly used preservation solutions

	EUROCOLLINS	UW	CELSIOR	HTK
Year		1987	1994	1975
Source		Belzer (USA)	Pasteur-Merieus (France)	Bretschneider (Germany)
Electrolytes (mmol/l)				
Na^+	10	25–30	100	15
K^+	115	125	15	10
Mg^{2+}	4	5	13	4
Ca^{2+}	–	–	0.25	0.015
Preventors of I-R injury				
Mannitol (g/l)	31	–	60	30
Glutathione (mmol/l)	–	3	3	–
Allopurinol (mmol/l)	–	1	–	1
Colloids				
HES (g/l)	–	50	–	–

Impermeants and Buffers (mmol/l)

Glucose	180	—	—	—
Lactobionic acid	—	100	80	—
Raffinose	—	30	—	—
Histidine	—	—	30	180
HCO_3	10	—	—	—
H_2PO_4/HPO_4	60	25	—	—
ATP precursors (mmol/l)				
Adenosine	—	5	—	—
Aminoglutaminic acid	—	—	20	—
Acetone dicarboxylic acid	—	—	—	1
Membrane stabilisation				
Tryptophan (mmol/l)	—	—	—	2

(continued)

TABLE 1.9 (continued)

	EUROCOLLINS	UW	CELSIOR	HTK
Additives to add				
Dexamethasone (mg/l)	–	16	–	–
Penicillin G (units/l)	–	200,000	–	–
Regulr Insulin (units/l)	–	40	–	–
pH	7.30	7.40	7.30	7.20
mOsmL/kg	340	320	320	310

Additional disadvantage of UW is its high viscosity (potential effect on microcirculation and therefore increase in biliary comlipications), high potassium content that may induce vasospasm and its price.

Other strategies include caspase inhibitors and perfluorocarbons (increase oxygen availability).

∗∗Current literature review:

(a) *The University of Wisconsin solution is the standard criterion static cold preservation for the procurement of liver, kidney, pancreas, and intestine. University of Wisconsin, HTK, and Celsior solutions all provide similar allograft outcomes in most clinical trials.*

(b) *Kidneys: UW and HTK have lower rates of DGF than Eurocollins.*

(c) *Pancreas: All three preservation solutions seem to perform equally well with shorter ischemia times (<12 h). There remains controversy regarding both Celsior solution and HTK solution with longer ischemia times, whereas University of Wisconsin solution seems to perform well even for more than 24 h of preservation.*

(d) *Liver: University of Wisconsin (UW) solution has been recognized as the gold standard in liver preservation, but its limitations are becoming obvious, such as risk of biliary complications and its high cost. HTK was thought to be more effective for biliary tract flush and prevention of biliary complications in some studies. There was no statistically significant difference of effects (except bile production) between HTK and UW. But trends were documented in some studies for the superiority of HTK in biliary tract flush, prevention of biliary complications, and cost saving.*

(c) **Machine perfussion**: given the shortage of donors worldwide, continuous perfusion of donor organs through machine pump with use of preservation solutions could increase the donor pool. The use of marginal organs has also turned the atention into the preservation related ischaemia-reperfusion injury. This injury is probably the most important factor that influences graft dysfunction.

Attenuation of this factor and resuscitation of the graft with continuous circulation of energy substrates and washout of waste products is possible with the use of these new ex vivo preservation techniques. Also, this new machines will let the transplant team to have an assessment of tissue metabolism and viability, through measurement of preservation fluid parameters.

- Hypothermic machine perfusion (HMP):
  - Hypothermia reduces aerobic respiration and therefore celular insults by keeping provision of high-energy metabolic substrate. The continuous perfusion of the liver improves the dilution and washout of toxic metabolites and waste products.
  - Kidneys with HMP have lower incidence of DGF. However there is still some controversy regarding long-term survival and patient survival rates.
  - Liver with HMP have decreased arteriolosclerosis in the peribiliary vascular plexus, increased O_2 uptake capacity and increased arterial flow after reperfusion.
  - There is the potencial for increase in graft and patient survival if HMP were applied in the clinical setting, although there are no long-term data available to make that statement.

- Normothermic machine perfusion: with this machine oxigenation is also possible, allowing restoration of normal aerobic metabolism and gives the possibility of a continuous assessment. Added to all these advantages, pharmacological modulation can be performed. It is based in a fully-cannulated circuit blood-based perfusate in which nutrition and key additives are infused with physiological pressures, flows and temperature.

  Reported from laboratory studies it seem to improve ability of organs to be used safely and reliably, providing better outcomes in liver function and histologic integrity when compared with cold storage.

More recents studies have showed lower incidence of intrahepatic biliary strictures, anastomotic biliary strictures and anastomotic biliary leaks.

- Normothermic Regional Perfusion: this technique is an in situ perfusion of abdominals organs using extracorporeal oxygenation using a membrane oxygenator, a heater and a pump. It is used to limits warm ischaemia by restoring the circulation before organ removal, allowing time for recovery of function and arresting and reversing depletion of ATP. This perfusion may increase the tolerance to cold ischaemia possibly by acting as a preconditioning stimulus.

(d) **Protective techniques:**

(a) Ischaemic precondition. Complex mechanism involving adenosin and nitric oxide released after short periods of ischaemica followed by reperfusion. This mechanism may ameliorate the hypoxic damage and improve the microcirculation (vasodilatation effect from NO and reduction in neutrophil accumulation).

(b) Pharmacological modulation (cytokine modulation, nitric oxide metabolism, prostaglandins, aminoacids, antioxidant therapy…).

1.3.6   Reception of the Tissue/Cells at the Tissue Establishment

- When the retrieved tissues/cells arrive at the tissue centre, there must be documented verification that the consignment, including the transport conditions, packaging, labelling and associated documentation and samples, meet the previous requirements and the specifications of the receiving establishment.
- Each centre must ensure that the tissue and cells received are quarantined until they, along with the associated documentation, have been inspected or otherwise verified as conforming to requirements. The review of relevant donor/

procurement information and thus acceptance of the donation needs to be carried out by specified/authorised persons.

1.4   Additional Professional Skills for the Retrieval Surgeon

Main aim of the full process of organ procurement is the harvesting of good quality organs for the purpose of transplantation. The retrieval surgeon needs to keep this in mind at all time understanding that the process is not only a surgical intervention but a very complex procedure involving multiple teams and factors. The surgeon is expected to behave as team leader since he will be responsible of the good ending of the donation.

Donation will take place in transplant centers but also in non-transplant ceters where theatre staff might not be used to this situation and this can lead into conflict. The retrieval team will act then as embassador of the transplant community as it is therefore of the greates importance that side skills, others that the surgical capacity, are considered. Good communication skills, teamwork and abilitiy to act in a multi-disciplinary enviroment are essentials.

The procurement surgeon must warranty that the enviroment is safe for the donor and staff and that the donor and relatives are treated respectfully. It is important to explain in detail to every member of the team that is going to be involved what is the plan and what are the expected steps. Being polite and approachable is important in order to clarify any doubt before the procedure start so everyone works in the same direction.

1.5   Ethics in Transplantation

Organ donation and transplantation are broad areas of medicine in which many ethical principles are in constant debate.

1.5.1 Organ Shortage (Limited Resources)

- There are more people on the waiting list than donated organs.
- The following information from UNOS gives an idea of the extent of the organ shortage:
  - "On average, 106 people are added to the nation's organ transplant waiting list each day--one every 14 min.
  - "On average, 68 people receive transplants every day from either a living or deceased donor.
  - "On average, 17 patients die every day while awaiting an organ – one person every 85 min.

1.5.2 Allocation Systems

- It is clear that the demand for an organ far outweighs the supply and therefore some allocation system is required.
- There is not one "right" way to distribute organs, but rather many ways a person could justify giving an organ to one particular individual over someone else.
- There are different principles used to solve the problem of scarce resources. Equity, utility and justice are some of them.
- Justice is the moral principle maintening of what is right or due to a person. This principle includes distributive justice (how to fairly divide resources through a given population) and compensatory justice (how individuals are compensated for efforts they have expended or harm they have suffered). With distributive justice, each patient waiting for an organ should recieve a fair chance at transplantation. With compensatory justice, a patient who agrees to accept a suboptimal organ, should receive some advantage (i.e.: quicker access to an organ).

- Utility tries to achieve the maximal benefits for a resource (survival in the case of transplantation). However the application of this principle does not account for those patients who do not receive the transplant and remain on the waiting list. Therefore, maximum benefit (measured by the total number of years gained) has been suggested as a better principle because it balances the risk of death on the waiting list and the post-transplant survival.
- Equal access to transplantation encourages an allocation system free of biases based on geographics and demographics factors of the patient. To fully achieve this principle is also required that patients with similar degree of illness, have the same probability of receiving an organ.

1.5.3   Donation after Brain Death

Although neurological determination of death is nearly worldwide accepted, uniformity in standards is not a rule. The possibility of declaring a person dead in one country and alive in another is still there.

Different cultures and religions make this need, even more difficult due to some societies and countries do not accept brain death as many strict Orthodox Jewish rabbis or some Islamic believers.

1.5.4   Donation after Circulatory Death

Apart of the obvious ethical issues of withdrawing supportive treatment in a dying patient, wait till is dead and retrieve his/her organs, there are two main ethical problems that are currently very highlighted. The first one is the duration of the time between asystolia and death confirmation. Some authors argue that is imposible to claim that there is an irreversible cessation of circulation and respiration. The important point is to differentiate between "irreversible" and "permanent". An irreversible cessation means that circulation will not return even using available technology. On the other hand, a permanent cessation means that circulation will not restart again because auto-resuscitation will not happen and because medical effort will not be done due to the patient has a Do-Not-Attempt-Resuscitation order. In controlled DCD patients where a cardiac arrest follows a respiratory arrest, no case of true auto-resuscitation has ever been reported, but there are well-described cases of auto-resuscitation in the literature in patients with cardiac arrest and subsequent respiratory arrest with unsuccessful CPR and death declaration. Given this fact, uncontrolled DCD patients are still an ethical problem.

The second controversy is the use of different medical technology and interventions on the donor in order to improve the organ perfusion and to avoid long warm ischamic time. The problem with the use of this devices as ECMO, is that its use could perfuse the brain and invalidate the death declaration. Therefore a balloon in the thoracic aorta is inflatted to avoid any blood flow to the brain.

Added to these concerns, some ethicists think that donation after circulatory death could be the first stept toward euthanasia. In fact, this kind of donations is not allowed in some countries.

1.5.5   The Dead Donor Rule

This well known axiom provides that in the context of transplantation organs should be removed from donors only when they are dead. This has been accepted for many years and has been crucial to maintain the confidence in physicians and the integrity of the donation practice. However some authors as Truog and Miller argue that this rule should be replaced, claiming that a voluntary donation in an ill patient should be enough to permit donation without requiring that the donor be dead.

Bibliography

1. Abdominal Perfusion and Preservation Protocol for NORS Teams in the UK. NHSBT. https://nhsbtdbe.blob.core.windows.net/umbraco-assets-corp/1403/abdominal_perfusion_protocol.pdf.
2. Aulisio MP, Devita M, Luebke D. Taking values seriously: ethical challenges in organ donation and transplantation for critical care professionals. Crit Care Med. 2007;35(2 Suppl):S95–101.
3. Ausania F, Drage M, Manas D, Callaghan CJ. A registry analysis of damage to the deceased donor pancreas during procurement. Am J Transplant. 2015;15(11):2955–62.
4. Balfoussia D, Yerrakalva D, Hamaoui K, Papalois V. Advances in machine perfusion graft viability assessment in kidney, liver, pancreas, lung, and heart transplant. Exp Clin Transplant. 2012;10(2):87–100.
5. Benamu E, Wolfe CR, Montoya JG. Donor-derived infections in solid organ transplant patients: toward a holistic approach. Curr Opin Infect Dis. 2017;30(4):329–39. https://doi.org/10.1097/QCO.0000000000000377.
6. Bernat JL. How can we achieve uniformity in brain death determinations? Neurology. 2008;70:252–3.
7. Bernat JL. How auto-resuscitation impacts death determinations in organ donors. Crit Care Med. 2010;38:1377–8.
8. Brockmann JG, Vaidya A, Reddy S, Friend PJ. Retrieval of abdominal organs for transplantation. Br J Surg. 2006;93(2):133–46.
9. Cameron AM, Barandiaran Cornejo JF. Organ preservation review: history of organ preservation. Curr Opin Organ Transplant. 2015;20(2):146–51. https://doi.org/10.1097/MOT.0000000000000175.
10. Ceresa CDL, Nasralla D, Jassem W. Normothermic machine preservation of the liver: state of the art. Curr Transplant Rep. 2018;5(1):104–10. https://doi.org/10.1007/s40472-018-0186-9. Epub 2018 Feb 27
11. Ceresa CDL, Nasralla D, Knight S, Friend PJ. Cold storage or normothermic perfusion for liver transplantation: probable application and indications. Curr Opin Organ Transplant. 2017;22(3):300–5. https://doi.org/10.1097/MOT.0000000000000410.
12. Choinski K, Rocca JP, Torabi J, Lorenzen K, Yongue C, Herbert ME, Block T, Chokechanachaisakul A, Kamal L, Kinkhabwala M, Graham JA. The pancreas can take the cold: lower waitlist

times through importation. Transplant Proc. 2017;49(10):2305–9. https://doi.org/10.1016/j.transproceed.2017.10.006.

13. Completion Guidelines for Retrieval Team Information. NHSBT. https://nhsbtdbe.blob.core.windows.net/umbraco-assets-corp/12779/completion-guidelines-for-retrieval-team-information-rti-forms.pdf.

14. DuBose J, Salim A. Aggressive organ donor management protocol. J Intensive Care Med. 2008;23(6):367–75.

15. Feng S, Goodrich NP, Bragg-Gresham JL, Dykstra DM, Punch JD, DebRoy MA, Greenstein SM, Merion RM. Characteristics associated with liver graft failure: the concept of a donor risk index. Am J Transplant. 2006;6(4):783–90.

16. Findings During Retrieval Requiring Histopathology Assessment. NHSBT. https://nhsbtdbe.blob.core.windows.net/umbraco-assets-corp/6500/sop5352-findings-during-retrieval-requiring-histopathology-assessment.pdf.

17. Fischer SA. Is this organ donor safe?: Donor-Derived Infections in Solid Organ Transplantation. Surg Clin North Am. 2019;99(1):117–28. https://doi.org/10.1016/j.suc.2018.09.009.

18. Flores A, Asrani SK. The donor risk index: a decade of experience. Liver Transpl. 2017;23(9):1216–25. https://doi.org/10.1002/lt.24799.

19. Foley DP, Fernandez LA, Leverson G, Anderson M, Mezrich J, Sollinger HW, D'Alessandro A. Biliary complications after liver transplantation from donation after cardiac death donors: an analysis of risk factors and long-term outcomes from a single center. Ann Surg. 2011;253(4):817–25. https://doi.org/10.1097/SLA.0b013e3182104784.

20. Form for the Diagnosis of Death using Neurological Criteria. NHSBT. https://www.ficm.ac.uk/sites/default/files/Form%20for%20the%20Diagnosis%20of%20Death%20using%20Neurological%20Criteria%20-%20Full%20Version%20%282014%29.pdf.

21. Fridell JA, Mangus RS, Thomas CM, Kubal CA, Powelson JA. Donation after circulatory arrest in pancreas transplantation: a report of 10 cases. Transplant Proc. 2017;49(10):2310–4. https://doi.org/10.1016/j.transproceed.2017.10.009.

22. Furton EJ. Brain death, the soul, and organic life. Natl Cathol Bioeth Q. 2002;2:455–70.

23. Greenwald MA, Kuehnert MJ, Fishman JA. Infectious disease transmission during organ and tissue transplantation. Emerg Infect Dis. 2012;18(8):e1. https://doi.org/10.3201/eid1808.120277.

24. Greer DM, Varelas PN, Haque S, et al. Variability of brain death determination guidelines in leading US neurologic institutions. Neurology. 2008;70:284–9.
25. Hameed AM, Wong G, Laurence JM, Lam VWT, Pleass HC, Hawthorne WJ. A systematic review and meta-analysis of cold in situ perfusion and preservation for pancreas transplantation. HPB (Oxford). 2017;19(11):933–43. https://doi.org/10.1016/j.hpb.2017.07.012.. Epub 2017 Aug 24
26. Hosgood SA, van Heurn E, Nicholson ML. Normothermic machine perfusion of the kidney: better conditioning and repair? Transpl Int. 2015;28(6):657–64. https://doi.org/10.1111/tri.12319.. Epub 2014 May 8
27. Hornby K, Hornby L, Shemie SD. A systematic review of autoresuscitation after cardiac arrest. Crit Care Med. 2010;38:1246–53.
28. Institute of Medicine. Non-heart-beating organ transplantation: practice and protocols. Washington DC: National Academy Press; 2000.
29. Jenkins DH, Reilly PM, Schwab CW. Improving the approach to organ donation: a review. World J Surg. 1999;23(7):644–9.
30. Laurence JM, Cattral MS. Techniques of pancreas graft salvage/indications for allograft pancreatectomy. Curr Opin Organ Transplant. 2016;21(4):405–11. https://doi.org/10.1097/MOT.0000000000000318.
31. Fridell JA, Mangus RS, Chen JM, Taber TE, Cabrales AE, Sharfuddin AA, Yaqub MS, Powelson JA. Steroid-free three-drug maintenance regimen for pancreas transplant alone: comparison of induction with rabbit antithymocyte globulin +/− rituximab. Am J Transplant. 2018;18(12):3000–6.
32. Jun H, Jung CW, Lim S, Kim MG. Kidney donor risk index as the predictor for the short-term clinical outcomes after kidney transplant from deceased donor with acute kidney injury. Transplant Proc. 2017;49(1):88–91. https://doi.org/10.1016/j.transproceed.2016.11.003.
33. Manara AR, Murphy PG, O'Callaghan G. Donation after circulatory death. Br JAnaesthesia. 2012;108(suppl_1):i108–21.
34. Mascia L, Mastromauro I, Viberti S, Vincenzi M, Zanello M. Management to optimize organ procurement in brain dead donors. Minerva Anestesiol. 2009;75(3):125–33.. Epub 2008 Jan 24
35. Miller FG, Truog RD. Rethinking the ethics of vital organ donation. Hast Cent Rep. 2008;38:38–46.

36. McKeown DW, Bonser RS, Kellum JA. Management of the heartbeating brain-dead organ donor. Br J Anaesth. 2012;108(suppl_1):i96–i107.
37. Organ procurement and transplantation network policies. UNOS. https://optn.transplant.hrsa.gov/media/1200/optn_policies.pdf#nameddest=Policy_02.
38. Rao F, Yang J, Gong C, Huang R, Wang Q, Shen J. Systematic review of preservation solutions for allografts for liver transplantation based on a network meta-analysis. Int J Surg. 2018;54(Pt A):1–6. https://doi.org/10.1016/j.ijsu.2018.04.024. Epub 2018 Apr 21.
39. Rosner F. The definition of death in Jewish law. In: Youngner SJ, Arnold RM, Schapiro R, editors. The definition of death:contemporary controversies. Baltimore: Johns Hopkins University Press; 1999. p. 210–21.
40. Shemie SD, Baker AJ, Knoll G, et al. National recommendations for donation after cardiocirculatory death in Canada. CMAJ. 2006;175.(8 Suppl:S1–S24.
41. Truog RD, Miller FG. The dead donor rule and organ transplantation. N Engl J Med. 2008;359:674–5.

Chapter 2
Kidney Transplantation

Mohammad Ayaz Hossain, Radhika Chadha, Atul Bagul, and Reza Motallebzadeh

2.1 Introduction

Kidney transplantation has been the definitive treatment for end stage renal disease for the last 70 years. The fundamental principles of vascular anastomoses have been developed over the last one hundred years following the first recorded

———

M. A. Hossain
Department of Nephrology and Transplantation,
Royal Free Hospital, London, UK

R. Chadha
Department of Academic Surgery, Oxford University Hospital,
Oxford, UK

A. Bagul
Department of Renal Transplantation, Leicester General Hospital,
Leicester, UK

R. Motallebzadeh (✉)
Department of Nephrology and Transplantation,
Royal Free Hospital, London, UK

Division of Surgery and Interventional Sciences;
Centre for Transplantation, Department of Renal Medicine;
and Institute of Immunity and Transplantation,
University College London, London, UK
e-mail: r.motallebzadeh@ucl.ac.uk

© Springer Nature Switzerland AG 2019   69
R. Díaz-Nieto (ed.), *Procurement and Transplantation of Abdominal Organs in Clinical Practice*, In Clinical Practice,
https://doi.org/10.1007/978-3-030-21370-1_2

attempt at renal transplantation in 1902 in which a carotid to renal artery anastomosis was successfully accomplished. The use of the iliac vein and artery for renal transplantation, as pioneered by French surgeon Alex Carrel, still provides the foundations of the anastomotic technique utilised today. More recent advances in the field include the use of alternative vessels for anastomosis, variation in implantation site, performing the operation as part of a multi-visceral procedure and the use of suboptimal grafts.

Current research efforts focus on the non-surgical components of organ transplantation: organ procurement, preservation and machine perfusion, development of tolerance-inducing protocols requiring little or no immunosuppression, identification of novel biomarkers to identify recipients at risk of graft loss, and regenerative medicine applications to model disease processes and allow drug testing for therapeutic efficacy as well as to potentially create, engineer or repair organs for transplantation. Continuous improvements in short-term graft patency has led to renal transplantation becoming the optimal treatment for end-stage renal disease, with one-year graft survival rates from living-related and deceased donors approaching 95% and 91% respectively. However, long-term graft survival outcomes remain less impressive, with chronic rejection and death with a functioning graft being the leading causes of late loss of renal allografts (more than 1 year after transplantation), resulting in an annual rate of loss of 3–5%. The ongoing demand for kidney transplantation is therefore exacerbated by graft failure and the need for re-transplantation.

Between 1960 and 1980 the estimated incidence for graft loss from surgical complications was up to 20%. These rates have dropped significantly since then but early detection, diagnosis and management of surgical complications are critical to further reduce patient morbidity, and potentially mortality, through graft loss. This chapter provides an overview of the existing surgical techniques employed in the field of kidney donation and transplantation along with some of the proposed updates to these procedures.

2.2   Pre Operative Work up

2.2.1   Living Kidney Donation

The options for live kidney donation in the UK have expanded over the last 10 years. Alongside the known related or unrelated direct and paired donation, altruistic donation, with or without direction, has seen an increase in incidence. The surgical work up for each donor remains the same and it is increasingly apparent that the need for short and long term follow up after donor nephrectomy should be prioritised. Patients are counselled for the risk of hypertension as well as the development of end stage renal disease, which at 0.5%, still remains substantially lower than that of the 3.2% risk of end-stage renal failure in the general population.

Identification of peri-operative risks should commence like with any elective procedure, with the donor health and medical history. Significant comorbidities contraindicate donation. Uncontrolled hypertension and diabetes with their associated risk to kidney function are also contraindicated given the increased risk of end stage diabetic nephropathy at 5 years being in the region of 25%. The associated risk of hypertension not only affects the anaesthetic risk but also the theoretical risk of hyperfiltration following nephrectomy, leading to hyperalbuminuria and progressive glomerulopathy. Malignancy and infection in the history of the donor does not absolutely contraindicate donation, but every effort must be made to exclude recurrent disease, mitigate risk and prevent transmission to the recipient.

Another often considered and subsequently managed risk is obesity. Worldwide rates of obesity are increasing, and the boundaries of acceptability of donor body mass index (BMI) are widening. The almost ubiquitous use of laparoscopic techniques over open surgery has enabled donors with BMIs of up to 35 kg/m^2 to be routinely considered for donation. That being said there is a greater risk of post-operative morbidity in the obese, and careful pre-operative assessment to exclude cardiovascular, respiratory and kidney disease is advised. Of note, obesity is now recognised as an independent risk factor for end-stage renal disease. The higher rates of postoperative analgesic requirements, increased atelectasis, pneumonia and venous thrombosis should be considered along with the higher incidence of wound complications. The consequence is a lengthier hospital stay and an increased recovery period. In order to mitigate these risks whilst expanding the potential live donor pool, established robotic donor nephrectomy from urological practise has been performed in both the live donor and the recipient with equivalent outcomes reported to laparoscopic counterparts.

All donors routinely have biochemical assessment of their kidney function, previous or active infections (e.g. serological screening for cytomegalovirus (CMV), Epstein Barr virus (EBV), Herpes Simplex virus (HSV), Hepatitis B (HBV) and C (HCV) viruses, Human Immunodeficiency Virus (HIV), and Human T-cell Leukemia Virus, Toxoplasma and Treponema) and haematology along with an electrocardiogram (ECG). Urinalysis for protein, blood, leucocytes with appropriate culture and microscopy is routinely undertaken. Outside of these tests, other analyses are performed at the discretion of the investigator depending on baseline results.

During the work up of the donor, it is essential to establish not only the anatomy and the vasculature of the donor kidneys, but also an assessment of the function must be made as well. Given serum creatinine can be influenced by muscle mass, dietary intake and nutritional status, measured glomerular filtration rate (GFR) using a reference GFR procedure is considered more accurate. Pre-donation GFR should be such that the predicted post-donation GFR remains within the gender and age-specific normal range within the donor's lifetime. Further to this, a DMSA or MAG 3 scan assessment of function should also be performed which should give an equal split function across the two kidneys. When renal function is normal but there is a significant (>10%) difference in function between the two kidneys, the kidney with lower function should be used for transplantation.

Anatomical anomalies such as cysts or potential tumours should be interrogated with either serial CT or ultrasound scans supported ideally by a specialist radiologist. Once potential malignant lesions are excluded it is then important to establish the vascular anatomy, which can be complex. This enables surgical planning and the anticipation of potential risks in the donor and the need for reconstruction before recipient implantation.

Most centres prefer to use the left kidney for living kidney donation as the renal vein is longer on this side, which is advantageous during implantation. Nevertheless, a single-centre randomised controlled trial has shown no differences between left- and right-sided donor nephrectomy in hospital stay, quality of life, donor and recipient complication rates, or graft survival. The presence of multiple renal arteries or veins does not increase the risk of thrombosis or impact short and long-term graft survival. Increased rates of urinary leaks have been described in particular when associated with a small polar artery owing to the theoretical supply of ureteric vasculature predominantly from the polar vessel. Multiple renal veins are present in 5–10% of donors. Most of the small calibre accessory renal veins can safely be ligated, but occasionally reconstruction to gain length of a short right renal vein maybe necessary.

2.2.2   Recipient Assessment

The initiation of chronic kidney disease and the timing of transplantation can impact on the subsequent patient and graft survival. Pre-emptive (prior to the start of renal replacement therapy), offers a better quality of life for the patient with improved cardiovascular comorbidity risk post transplantation. Transplantation of the recipient within 6 months of requiring renal replacement therapy is the ideal standard. The relatively shorter cold and warm ischaemia times, coupled with the healthier donor (due to extensive pre-donation work-up), confer both short and long term survival advantage over the deceased donor counterpart. Nevertheless, not all recipients have this option. Waiting times for patients on the deceased waiting list average at 3 years in the UK and vary according to the recipients ABO blood group and calculated HLA antibody reaction frequency (CRF). It is therefore generally agreed that all recipients should have at least a cursory inquiry into the possibility of a potential live donor at the onset of waiting list assessment.

Outcome goals of the assessment of the transplant recipient are listed in Box 2.1.

Box 2.1 Outcome Goals for the Kidney Transplant Recipient. (Adapted from the UK Renal Association Kidney Transplant Guidelines, 5th Edition, 2010)

Goals of the Multidisciplinary Recipient Workup

- Ensure transplantation is technically possible;
- Ensure the recipient's chances of survival are not compromised by transplantation;
- Ensure that graft survival is not limited by premature death (maximum benefit obtained from a limited resource)
- Ensure pre-existing conditions are not exacerbated by transplantation
- Identify measures to be taken to minimise peri- and post-operative complications. Inform patients of likely risks and benefits of transplantation

Even though in most cases, the technical aspects, i.e. the approach and anastomosis of the kidney transplant to the recipient, may be feasible, there are some technical barriers to consider as part of the work up. One of the main considerations is the BMI of the patient. Obesity with a BMI of over 30 kg/m^2 carries high rates of peri-operative morbidity (seromas, wound dehiscence, infections, hernias) and generally it is thought that the benefit of transplanting a patient with a BMI >40 kg/m^2 is outweighed by the risks. Other technical considerations include space for implantation which can be an issue in patients with polycystic kidney disease. Vascular considerations need to be addressed especially when encountering heavily calcified arteries in long standing diabetic recipients. Venous outflow is rarely an issue but previous DVT or a propensity for thrombosis in familial conditions should be addressed appropriately and an anticoagulation plan sought where necessary.

As stated in the summary Box 2.1, the medical evaluation of the recipient is a multi-disciplinary process, which focuses on the factors that are likely to influence the safety of the recipient whilst maintaining an optimal outcome for the patient and graft, and thus enables the best utilistaiton of the donor organ. Identification at the outset of absolute contraindications to transplantation is critical. These include active malignancies, certain active infections, severe unmodifiable non-renal diseases e.g. cardiac impairment, psychiatric disease that will impact ability of the patient to adhere to long-term immunosuppression therapy, and active substance abuse. Since the subsequent lifelong immunosuppression to be taken by the recipient will cause a higher risk of malignancy, the assessment of recurrent disease needs to be evaluated. The status of treatments for cervical, bladder, prostate, colonic and skin cancers should be ascertained although outcomes of transplantation after treatment of early stages of these cancers have shown to have good prognoses on registry data.

As the leading cause of death in patients with end-stage renal disease is cardiovascular related disease, the identification of risk factors that can be modified prior to transplantation is critical. A basic history should cover management of diabetes, hypertension, smoking, hyperlipidaemia and identify family history risk of coronary artery disease. Perioperative risks are increased with myocardial infarction 6 months prior to surgery, unstable angina, congestive heart failure and the onset of arrhythmias. Even though routine screening using stress echocardiography and exercise testing can be time consuming and expensive, their use in high risk or symptomatic recipients such as patients with diabetes can help permit operative prediction of the likely level of care (ward, high dependency or intensive care). Referral to a cardiology department for treatment of severe coronary artery occlusive disease is mandatory prior to transplantation.

All sources of bacterial infection should be identified during routine assessment. Areas to be considered include peritoneal catheter sites, dental abscesses, vascular access grafts along with routine urine dipsticks and cultures. Persistent urological infections should be further investigated with pyelography (CT or fluoroscopy) with ultrasound to ensure complete bladder emptying and where necessary cystoscopy.

Routine serology is common practise and recommended by the UK Renal association. This includes viral studies for IgG and IgM titres of CMV, EBV, HSV and Hepatitis and HIV viruses. The use of pan-genotypic direct antiviral agents is likely to mean that Hepatitis B and C donors are no longer contraindicated to use in non-Hepatitis B and C recipients; at present this practise is not universal.

Assessment of the recipient bladder function can be difficult in the anuric dialysis patient. This is often best left to post-transplantation when kidney function has stabilised. Screening early on in the assessment of elderly (over 60 year old) men for prostate disease with a documented digital rectal examination and a serum prostate specific antigen is often all that is required to identify those at risk. Diabetic patients often have neurogenic bladders that should be treated post-transplantation if high residual volumes are discovered after removal of the urinary catheter post-surgery. Patients with prior cystectomies that have ileal conduits or augmented bladder should be fully investigated with the aid of CT scanning and cystoscopy to delineate the appropriate anatomy prior to listing for transplantation. In this small subgroup of patients, a clear plan for bladder reconstruction or creation of a neocystoureterotomy should be documented.

2.3   Surgical Technique

2.3.1   Deceased Donor Procurement

Deceased kidney procurement occurs in sequence, following the other abdominal organs (namely liver and pancreas) in both donation after brain-death (DBD) and donation after circulatory death (DCD) donors.

There is a distinct warm phase in DBD donors, whereby careful exposure the inferior vena cava (IVC), left renal vein with mobilization of the duodenum in its entirety superiorly and laterally (Cattell-Braasch manoeuvre), is undertaken. Once key vessels are identified, including the superior mesenteric artery (SMA) caudal to the left renal vein crossing the aorta, the infra-renal aorta either proximal to its bifurcation or the common iliac artery can be cannulated to proceed to the cold phase.

The cold phase of procurement is very similar in both DBD and DCD procurement. Unlike DBD, there is no period of warm dissection in DCD and rapid cannulation of the aorta with either IVC or right atrial venting is undertaken through a midline sternotomy and laparotomy. Cross clamping of the aorta in both DBD and DCD procurement can either take place in the supra-coeliac position below the diaphragm, or (as is the authors preference) in the thoracic descending aorta. It is common to wait for 5 min in DBD procurement whilst an intravenous bolus of heparin 20–30,000 units is given to prevent thrombosis after cross-clamping. In DCD procurement, the cold perfusion fluid is normally heparinised with a similar amount. Optional back table perfusion should be prepared in case once the organs are inspected, perfusion is deemed inadequate.

After cold perfusion of the aorta has commenced, ice slush is applied to both paracolic gutters to commence topical cooling whilst the liver and pancreas are mobilised and removed. It should be noted that the plane between the right lobe of the liver and the right kidney should be dissected through the adrenal gland thus avoiding kidney or liver capsular injury. Similarly, on the left, a plane close to if not upon the left adrenal gland should be maintained to avoid pancreatic capsular or parenchymal injury.

Mobilisation of the colon should be swiftly undertaken commencing from the ileocolic junction to the descending aspect. Transection of the duodenal-jejunal junction should be performed with a linear stapling device which will allow division of the small bowel mesentery (again with multiple linear staples if pancreatic procurement is performed). Once this has been completed, the entire small bowel and colon can be exteriorised completely, allowing full view of the abdominal aorta. The left renal vein is then identified and finger swept underneath to allow a cuff of IVC to be taken when transected. Once the SMA is identified and divided at its base, the remaining aorta can be opened and split in the midline. The authors recommend a clean knife blade (size 10) in order to ensure precision in cutting the Carrel patch and avoiding injury to the renal artery ostia. At this point, the IVC can be divided superior to the right renal vein allowing enough renal vein for the recipient surgeon on both the liver and renal side. This is usually 2 finger breadths (1 cm) above the right renal vein.

The right renal ureter is identified first by encircling the peri-ureteric tissue commencing laterally from the psoas to the midline at the level of the right common iliac artery. Care should be taken to avoid removing the peri-ureteric tissue and cause "stripping of the ureter". The ureter should be accompanied by at least 1 cm of the peri-ureteral tissues and also the hilar inferior triangle (e.g. the window between the inferior pole of the graft and the ureteral origin from the renal pelvis) should be maintained intact. Once the ureter has been identified, the aortic patch can be mobilised posteriorly maintaining a close plane to the lumbar spine. The right kidney is mobilised by extending the existing plane of dissection towards the psoas, gently pulling the kidney medially. It is possible to apply a haemostat across the ureter at this point and transect the aortic patch and IVC inferiorly, thus releasing the kidney, although it is the authors' preference that both the aorta and IVC are transected free leaving the kidney on the ureteric pedicle as the last element to be divided before the organ is placed immediately on ice.

The left kidney is mobilised in a similar manner. The superior plane in the spleno-renal ligament should be carefully transected to avoid traction injury to the pancreas. Mobilisation of the left colon will have already occurred, and excessive traction of the colon, which can lead to inadvertent transection of the left main renal artery or a polar vessel, should be avoided. Retroperitoneal mobilisation is similar to that of the right kidney with transection of the aorta and iliac veins being recommended prior to the ureter.

After placement of the kidneys on ice, the circumferential fat along the lateral aspect of the kidney should be removed as much as possible. This facilitates both cooling of the organ and allows inspection for lesions, the general state of perfusion and any damage that may have occurred. The organ should then be triple bagged in cold storage fluid for transport.

2.3.2   Live Donor Nephrectomy

The first successful living donor kidney transplant originated in 1954 at the Peter Bent Brigham Hospital. Subsequently, due to the convenience of live donor implants over the logistical challenges of deceased donors, expansion of transplantation in non-identical twin pairs and then on to related non-twin siblings were favoured. By the mid 1960's and with the pioneering drive of Thomas Starzl, living donor transplantation in the USA was well established. Developmental progress in tissue typing and immunosuppression regimens was made by Paul Terasaki and colleagues to form the basis of modern protocols. It was not until 40 years after the first successful kidney transplant that a major technical step was made in procuring kidneys from live donors.

First described by Lloyd Ratner in 1995, laparoscopic donor nephrectomy was a major step in the surgical community in driving live-donor kidney transplantation. This has become the preferred method for procuring kidney grafts from living donors and accounts for over 90% of live donor nephrectomies performed in most high-volume transplane centres. Currently the options for laparoscopic donor nephrectomy are numerous, with both hand assisted and total laparoscopy assisting trans- or retro- peritoneal approaches (Box 2.2).

Box 2.2 Techniques in Living Donor Nephrectomy

Surgical techniques for living kidney donation

Open donor nephrectomy technique
  Classical flank incision
  Muscle-sparing mini-incision donor nephrectomy
Laparoscopic transperitoneal technique (∗)
  Laparoscopic donor nephrectomy
  Hand-assisted laparoscopic donor nephrectomy
Endoscopic retroperitoneal technique (∗)
  Endoscopic retroperitoneal donor nephrectomy
  Hand-assisted Endoscopic retroperitoneal donor nephrectomy

∗can also be performed with robotic assistance

Given the above work up of the live-donor with appropriate investigations, consent is obtained outlining the risks in the immediate, early and late operative phases. Potential injury to visceral structures around the kidney should be outlined necessitating the risk of conversion to an open procedure to repair the injury or control any bleeding. This may or may not impact on donation, in which case any event or injury deemed to impact permanently on the health of the donor may cease the process of donation in its entirety.

Donor nephrectomy is by convention performed in the lateral decubitus position. Therefore, the donor is warned of the risk of deep vein thrombosis, pulmonary embolus, peripheral nerve injury and back pain, with the former requiring the use of prophylactic low molecular weight heparin for up to 2 weeks post-surgery. In addition to this, the risk of hypertension in the donor should be explained along with the remote risk of developing renal failure in the remaining solitary kidney. Other risks commonly outlined to the donor are listed in Box 2.3.

Box 2.3 Common and Important Risks Associated with Laparoscopic Donor Nephrectomy

Potential risks of Laparoscopic Donor Nephrectomy

- Mortality range from 1 in 1600 to 1 in 2400
- Conversion to open procedure up to 2%
- Major risks (up to 5%)

  1. Bleeding
  2. Visceral injury
  3. DVT / PE
  4. Wound infection
  5. Chest complications- atelectasis, pneumonia
  6. Urinary tract infection
  7. Adhesions
  8. Wound pain, collections; incisional hernia

- General Anaesthesia risks
- Risks of living with a solitary kidney

  1. Hypertension
  2. Microscopic Haematuria
  3. End stage renal disease 0.9% plus requiring the need for renal replacement therapy if remaining kidney is removed for cancer or trauma

2.3.2.1   Laparoscopic Hand Assisted Donor Nephrectomy

By definition, the removal of a kidney for the purpose of allograft transplantation using both laparoscopy with the placement of a hand into the periotneal cavity/retroperitoneum is termed laparoscopic hand assisted donor nephrectomy. The ability of a silicone gel hand port enables the hand to be placed in the abdomen without loss of pneumoperitoneum (set at 12–15 mmHg). Both retroperitoneal and transperitoneal approaches have been described in the literature with excellent outcomes and acceptability to the donor. Ostensibly transperitoneal laparoscopic donor nephrectomy has been widely adopted over the retroperitoneal technique in part because most transplant and general surgeons are familiar with peritoneal insufflation and working within the peritoneal space.

With the patient supine, the first port is marked on the skin as the hand port, with the authors preference for this to be drawn just above the pubic symphisis along the "bikini line". It is ideal for this should to be drawn to the size of the operator's hand with the patient asleep, fully relaxed and supine, as the midline of the abdomen may shift during repositioning to the lateral decubitus position. Alternative sites for the hand port include a midline supraumbilical, periumbilical or infraumbilical incision. The hand port can be used partly or totally during the operation. A further 2 ports are introduced - a 12 mm port lateral to the umbilicus, and then under vision for the 30^0 camera, a 5 mm lateral port for the working instrument can be an used for an energy device or conventional diathermy. For the right kidney, an optional peri-xiphoid 5 mm port may be required to help retract the liver. The insufflation pressure is set maximally at 12 mmHg.

In the transperitoneal approach, the left or right colon is mobilised along the avascular white line of Toldt towards the pelvis. Gerota's fascia at this point is generally left in place, so that this does not fall and obscure the operators view. In order to expose the renal vein, the fascia overlying the vein is dissected and the renal vein identified. On the left, the adrenal and gonadal tributary is also identified. Gerota's fascia is divided over the adrenal gland at the upper pole, extending posteriorly and inferiorly to the spleen. Mobilisation of the adrenal gland is preferentially left before complete renal mobilisation as this area can inadvertently bleed.

The ureter and gonadal vein are usually identified inferiorly towards the pelvis and then traced back toward the kidney hilum. Digital sweeping of the tissue laterally with a finger around the gonadal vein and ureter permits mobilisation caudally. With the gonadal vein mobilised at least 2 cm away from the renal vein, it is ligated twice with a clip and then divided. This is then repeated in a similar manner for the adrenal vein approximately 1 cm at least away from the renal vein. Adequate length of the renal vein on the left side can often be attained without this manoeuvre and should not compromise risk of bleeding from an IVC cuff that retracts after ligation. With lumbar vessels draining into the renal vein identified and ligated, the renal artery can then be dissected by releasing the tissue around its base. This can be facilitated by posterior retroperitoneal release of the kidney, enabling anterior and posterior views of the renal artery. Once the kidney is mobile in this back and forth motion, the tissue between the renal artery and vein can be divided adequately to ensure passage of the linear cutting endostapling device. Once the ureter is divided with Hem-o-lok® clips and scissors, the vessels can then be divided. It is the authors preference to use a linear stapler (the authors preference is the Echelon Flex™ angulated stapler, Ethicon US) across the renal artery first and then the vein, although it is recognised that Ligaclips and plastic Hem-o-lok® clips have been utilised in centres outside the UK, with the advantage of millimetres of length gained on the organ vasculature. The counter to this is the catastrophic effect of a potential slip of clips/ligatures, with the ensuing morbidity or indeed mortality. Once divided, the mobile kidney can be removed via the hand port and handed to the recipient surgeon on ice to be cold perfused.

It is vitally important at this stage to remain focused on the donor, with the camera remaining inside to ensure no immediate bleeding. Both staple lines should be inspected after identification, with judicious haemostasis around the renal bed. The 12 mm port can be closed intracorporally and the Pfannenstiel hand port wound closed in a layered standard fashion with 1 Polydioxanone or Prolene suture. It is sometimes advocated in donors with an elevated BMI a closed suction drain applied to the wound to limit the development of seroma, although this observational practise is not supported with high level evidence.

The advantages of hand-assisted laparoscopic donor nephrectomy over full laparoscopy include the ability to use tactile feedback, less kidney traction, rapid control of bleeding, fast kidney removal, less blood loss and shorter warm ischaemic periods. The hand port provides additional safety to laparoscopic donor nephrectomy, because rapid control of potential massive blood loss from major blood vessels is possible with hand assistance. The disadvantage includes higher costs associated with a hand port, a worse ergonomic position for the surgeon during the operation, and a higher rate of wound infections.

2.3.2.2 Laparoscopic Retroperitoneal Donor Nephrectomy

By far the most common approach to the retroperitoneum for donor nephrectomy is with the use of a hand for assistance (HARS). As previously mentioned, the HARS technique confers the safety advantage by allowing immediate haemostasis should there be a severe sudden bleed. In a pure laparoscopic procedure, sudden severe bleeding from a major vessel is much harder to control and the necessity for open conversion is always prioritised. Other advantages are listed in Box 2.4.

Box 2.4 Advantages of Hand Assisted Retroperitoneal Donor Nephrectomy

<u>**Advantages of hand assisted and retroperitoneal nephrectomy over total laparosopic nephrectomy**</u>

1. Port placement- safer with the hand, reduced risk to visceral structures
2. Control of bleeding- immediate with the hand in abdominal cavity
3. Prevention of torsion of the kidney
4. No risk of internal herniation
5. Secure/Rapid placement of staplers
6. Secure/Rapid retrieval of the kidney
7. Reduction in warm ischaemia time
8. Shorter learning curve
9. Reduced risk of bowel obstruction
10. Reduced risk of adhesions and internal hernias

2.3.2.3   Fully Laparoscopic Donor Nephrectomy

Without the tactile sensation of the hand inside the abdomen, the approach to the fully laparoscopic donor nephrectomy is slightly more technically challenging than its hand assisted counterpart and has a steeper learning curve. Dissection of tissues is of critical importance and vigilance must be taken on both the retracting forceps as well as the working energy device dissection.

Port placement is again user dependant, but the authors agree on the common placement of a subxiphoid 5 mm port, a periumbilical 12 port, a lateral 12 mm port and a lower Pfannenstiel incision similar to the hand port of the hand assisted approach, measuring approximately 6–8 cm in diameter and lying approximately 1–2 cm above the pubic symphysis centred over the midline.

Mobilisation of the colon is performed in a similar fashion to that previously stated, with medial visceral rotation carefully performed to identify the ureter whilst separating the mesocolon from the mesoureteral structures in the avascular plane.

Identification of the ureter and dissection laterally over the psoas enables caudal mobilisation towards the renal pelvis and the kidney. In a similar manner to the hand assisted approach, careful identification of the gonadal and adrenal tributaries from the renal vein should be undertaken, with the former being traced from the ureteric pedicle. As previously stated, dissection around the hilum and identification of the renal artery can take place once the vein is in clear view. The adrenal vein tributary at the superior aspect of the renal vein can be isolated with a right-angled dissector, ligated and clipped before being transected.

It is the authors' preference to identify the plane between the adrenal gland and the kidney, and dissect close to the adrenal with electrocautery. Once the adrenal gland is separated, mobilisation towards the spleen can then take place with division of the splenorenal ligament using a Ligasure or similar device. The upper pole of the kidney will be fully mobile now, with the fat between the vessels remaining to be dissected. The latter should be done with great care so as not to cause traction injury to the renal artery. Once the posterior retroperitoneal attachments to the kidney are released and the vessels mobilised, stapling of the renal artery followed by the vein, in a similar manner to the hand assisted approach, can take place. An Endo Catch™ is inserted via the lower abdominal Pfannenstiel incision, with care taken to maintain the pneumoperitoneum by creating a purse string suture in the peritoneum before the instrument enters the abdominal cavity. Once the Endo Catch™ is removed with the kidney, the purse string can be pulled close to enable inspection of the renal bed for haemostasis along with identification of the staple lines.

2.3.2.4   Open Retroperitoneal Nephrectomy

In the era of laparoscopy, the open donor nephrectomy operation in the developed world has become largely historical. Having been the standard from 1954 until the mid 1990s, the operation is still performed in a minimal access manner in limited numbers, but has largely been replaced with the previously described minimally invasive techniques. Laparoscopic donor nephrectomy is associated with a significantly shorter hospital stay, fewer postoperative analgesic requirements, improved cosmetic appearance and a quicker return to work as compared with open donor nephrectomy and results in similar allograft function. The slight disadvantage of the laparoscopic technique is that it results in a shorter vascular pedicle when compared with the open donor nephrectomy. The warm ischaemia time and operating time for laparoscopic donor nephrectomy is also substantially longer than compared with open donor nephrectomy. A 2008 meta-analysis of 4 randomised control trials comparing laparoscopic with open donor nephrectomy found no significant difference in post-operative complications, although longer warm ischaemia times were noted in with the former.

With the patient positioned in the lateral decubitus position, an incision is conventionally made between the anterior superior iliac spine and the 12th rib anterior to the mid axillary line. Resection of the distal part of the lowest rib can be applied to allow sufficient access to the kidney. Dissection and division of the latissimus dorsi, external oblique, internal oblique and transversus abdominus muscles should occur with exposure of the peritoneum which can then be swept medially to enter into the retroperitoneum. Judicious retraction is required at this point to expose Gerota's fascia which can be divided to enable exposure of the kidney hilum. Once the perinephric fat is divided, the vessels can be easily identified and isolated with a vessel sling. The adrenal gland can be bluntly dissected with a finger with cautious use of electrocautery to ensure minimal bleeding. Once the vessels are isolated and the tributaries ligated, adequate artery and vein length should be obtained in order to pass a haemostat across their respective bases. The vascular pedicles are oversewn with 5–0 Prolene suture. Once divided, the ureter can be identified on its pedicle and transected with adequate length using a Hem-o-lok® clip and scissors.

With one of the most common post-operative complications from open nephrectomy being incisional hernias, judicious haemostasis and layered closure should take place in a systematic and precise fashion. Each muscle layer is closed with a 1 Polydiaxanone suture and the deep dermal layer approximated with 3–0 Vicryl absorbable suture. It is not the authors preference not to leave a drain unless there is an absolute necessity or the risk of seroma formation e.g. in high BMI (>35 kg/m^2) patients.

2.3.2.5   Robotic Donor Nephrectomy

Robotic surgery in donor nephrectomy was first reported in 2002. Use of a multi-armed, multi-port instrument with the operating surgeon in a separate operating module is now widely established in urological practise. The application in transplantation not only in donor nephrectomy but also in recipient implantation has gained much momentum over the last decade with leading centres in India and the USA publishing case series. The potential advantages sought over conventional laparoscopy lies in the optics and dexterity the arms of the robotic instruments can provide.

The donor nephrectomy is performed with the patient in a decubitus position. Four trocars are placed in the left or right side of the abdomen to allow placement of three articulated robotic arms, the robotic camera, and the standard laparoscopic instruments used for retraction and dissection during the procedure.

The limitation of laparoscopic instruments is their inability to articulate fine dissection of hilar vessels in a confined space. This is where the use of the small multi-faceted robotic arms excels. Proponents of the technique claim the potential to create vascular exposure and increase length of vessels working in a limited space. There is also the potential reduction in dissection time in the skilled operators hands, although the authors find limited published evidence for this. Whether this level of finesse impacts on graft outcome is again not evidenced. Currently, for many units the high costs of the machine and consumables makes the technology a non-essential commodity. Nonetheless despite longer operating times and warm ischaemia, post-operative pain requirements are reportedly reduced in donors without impact on immediate function.

2.3.2.6   Donor's Complications

Both laparoscopic and open donor nephrectomy operations potentially have significant operative risks that should be outlined at the time of consenting. Registry data has found that the mean stay after laparoscopic donor nephrectomy to be approximately 2.5 days with the quoted overall complication rate to be between 6–8%, whereas for open nephrectomy the mean length of stay is 5 days with an overall quoted complication rate of 2%. The 90-day mortality rate after laparoscopic and open nephrectomy is 0.03% and 0.04% respectively. The main significant difference is the return to work and normal activity, which is on average 6 weeks after laparoscopy and can be up to 3 months following open donation. Major complications (Clavien grade ≥ 3), are rare, ranging from 3 to 6%, with the overall rate of morbidity significantly higher after open donor nephrectomy compared to laparoscopic nephrectomy.

One of the most important potential risks is the development of end stage renal disease (ESRD) following kidney donation and has been quoted as low as 0.9% over 15 years. Even though this risk remains higher, however, than matched non-donor counterparts, it remains much less than that of the general (unscreened) population. Compared to the general public, kidney donors have equivalent (or better) survival, excellent quality of life, and no increase in ESRD. Certain patient groups (e.g. Afro-Caribbean donors, younger donors, genetically related donors, donors to patients with immunological causes of renal failure, and overweight donors) have a higher risk of ESRD following donation.

For the recipient, the benefits of living, compared to deceased-donor, kidney transplantation are well known with most donors also enjoying a quality of life that is similar or even better when compared with the general population. These results are linked to the intense medical evaluation of potential donors, resulting in the selection of only healthy and motivated individuals. Several studies have reported a better quality of life of donors after laparoscopic donor nephrectomy than after open donor nephrectomy, and in terms of costs, although laparoscopic donor nephrectomy has the potential to be more expensive due to the use of disposable instruments, better cost-effectiveness has been found compared with open donor nephrectomy.

2.3.3   Recipient Implantation

The basic operative methodology for renal transplantation has changed little from the principles of vascular anastomosis described by Alexis Carrel in 1902 and subsequently revised by René Küss and colleagues in 1951. Preparation and preservation of the kidney is essential to maximise early and late graft function after transplantation and is achieved in part through the use of preservation solutions and maintaining the graft in hypothermic conditions.

Three approaches exist with regard to the surgical placement of the renal allograft: (1) extraperitoneal, (2) transperitoneal, and (3) intraperitoneal. Traditionally implantation has been extraperitoneal in the iliac fossa for renal transplantation alone or a simultaneous liver-kidney transplant owing to the superficial position of the external iliac vein and ease of graft assessment by palpation and biopsy. For a a simultaneous pancreas-kidney transplant, the left iliac fossa is preferred for the renal allograft as this will allow for implantation of the pancreas the right side, with pancreas exocrine drainage via the small bowel or bladder and endocrine release into the systemic circulatory system via the IVC or common iliac vein. A transperitoneal approach may be used following failed kidney transplants in both iliac fossae and the intraperitoneal approach in small children to accommodate the relatively large graft. Morbidity associated with an intraperitoneal approach remains higher than extraperitoneal, with complications such as visceral injury or bowel obstruction and adhesions almost exclusively observed in the former. In the case of dual kidney transplantation (DKT), these are often split for individual implantation either ipsilaterally or bilaterally in the iliac fossae of the recipient via a classic Rutherford Morrison incision and will be discussed in more detail below.

2.3.3.1   Implantation Site

As alluded to above, the classical site for renal transplantation is the right iliac fossa, centred over the external iliac vasculature, as the longer and more horizontal right external iliac vessels facilitate easier vascular anastomoses. However, the advantage of placing the donor kidney in the recipient's contralateral side ensures the renal pelvis and ureter lie anterior and will be easier to access should the need arise for further surgeries (e.g. ureteric reconstruction). Other factors to consider when deciding on the site of surgery include previous surgery (e.g. failed renal transplantation), severe atherosclerotic/calcific disease affecting iliac arteries, and previous pelvic exploration and peritoneal dialysis catheters and are further outlined in Table 2.1. The use of both internal iliac arteries in serial renal transplantations in men is avoided to prevent impotence. Large grafts have historically been implanted within the abdominal cavity so as to prevent potential "kidney compartment" syndrome (over compression of the renal parenchyma limiting venous outflow). However it is the authors preference to still place the large kidney allograft into the iliac fossa but use either a subrectus pouch to position the kidney, a mesh to enable fascial closure without compression or use the right iliac retroperitoneal space to permit dital aortic anastomosis or common iliac artery with venous drainage either to the inferior vena cava or common iliac vein.

TABLE 2.1 Factors to take into consideration for implantation site

Factor	Preferred Site	Explanation
Previous surgeries	Opposite iliac fossa	Prevention of visceral/vessel injury or lymphocele and shorter operative time
Multivisceral operation	Left iliac fossa in the retroperitoneal space Abdominal cavity for en bloc Paediatric transplantation	Prevention of complications spreading from one graft to another
Size/length/number of graft arteries and veins	Iliac fossa	Prevention of postoperative ileus
Size/length/number of ureters	Iliac fossa if recipient ureter not diseased	Prevention of urine leakage or ureteral stricture
Number of kidney grafts	Retroperitoneal space of right iliac fossa	In this case it is better may be better to use the abdominal aorta/common iliac artery and inferior vena cava
Anomalies of donor graft	Abdominal cavity/iliac fossa depending on size of graft	Space consideration for graft and anastomotic sites for graft vessels/ureters

Historically, the three incisions used for renal transplantation are the Gibson incision, the 'hockey stick' incision and the Rutherford Morrison oblique incision. The Gibson incision is the most common approach and involves a relatively atraumatic curvilinear incision that starts two centimetres medially to the anterior superior iliac spine, running 0.5 centimetres above the inguinal fold, and is continued to the lateral border of the rectus muscle. The para-rectus 'hockey stick' incision is prolonged medially to the midline above the pubic symphysis and can be extended upward to the subcostal margin. One advantage of this approach is that it yields better access to the common iliac vessels and inferior vena cava. Its disadvantages include denervation of the para-rectal groove, lesser strength of abdominal wall closure, and potentially inferior cosmetic appearance due to its direction against the Langer's skin lines. Although shorter in length, the oblique incision may require the division of all the lateral abdominal muscles. Nanni and colleagues compared the 'hockey stick' and oblique incisions for post-operative complications and concluded that the latter was associated with a reduced incidence of incisional hernia and achieved a more favourable cosmetic appearance. Whichever approach is used, it is imperative that all incisions are accompanied by strict haemostasis to avoid wound or peri-graft haematomas that could eventually lead to infection, dehiscence, kidney compartment syndrome from compression of the graft.

Mobilization of a length of the external iliac vessels is subsequently conducted (and common iliac arteries is also needed when the internal iliac artery is considered as the candidate of arterial anastomosis). Exposure of the iliac vessels requires precise technique to avoid peritoneal injury and enteroceles, commonly described as a 'renal paratransplant hernia'. In addition, post-renal transplant lymphoceles resulting from inadequate lymphatic ligation can result in unnecessary patient morbidity. One study that followed up the impact of surgical technique on the incidence of lymphoceles reported that thorough ligation of all lymphatics using silk ties, both during dissection of the recipient vessels and the donor allograft, significantly reduces the incidence of this complication (with only one patient in their series of 273 transplants developing a lymphocele).

Following iliac vessel mobilization, the process of vascular anastomosis begins after choosing suitable points of vascular inflow and outflow along the iliac vessels. The site of each anastomosis and the position of the graft should be specified accurately according to the size and length of the vessels and also the length of the ureter and position of the recipient bladder. The kidney graft is placed in the wound and the renal vessels stretched to the recipient vessels to determine the best sites for the arterial and venous anastomoses. After confirming the exact length and position of the anastomosis site to prevent donor vessel kinking or rotation, vascular clamps are applied to the recipient vessels. We prefer to use Statinsky clamps for side-clamping of the external iliac vein or inferior vena cava and angled Dardik clamps to the common or external iliac artery.

It is important the anastomosis steps are completed carefully but in a timely manner as the kidney lies outside the body (i.e. out of cold storage) for this process, thus theoretically presenting an opportunity for warm ischaemic graft insult. The classical technique involves end-to-side venous anastomosis first, followed by an end-to-side arterial anastomosis.

2.3.3.2   Venous Anastomoses

Classically, allograft renal vein to the recipient iliac vein is anastomosed in an end-to-side fashion using a continuous monofilament suture (5–0 or 6–0 Prolene). The venous valve site in the external iliac vein should be avoided, if possible, as the wall of the vein is very thin proximal to the venous valves (sinuses of Valsalva) and may be ruptured during the anastomosis. The length of the donor vein of a right kidney can be increased by refashioning the inferior vena cava cuff which may be of particular importance in a short right renal vein (Fig. 2.1). Saphenous, gonadal or superficial femoral vein grafts as well as polytetrafluoroethylene grafts have also been used to successfully elongate short donor veins. It is the authors opinion that venous reconstruction is probably best avoided when using kidneys with prolonged cold ischemic times and from DCD donors to avoid the risk of venous thrombosis. Any reconstructions of the donor vein should take place prior to implantation of the kidney and, as mentioned below, excessive elongation should be avoided to protect against renal vein kinking and thrombosis; this is particular true for the left renal vein which is invariably shortened.

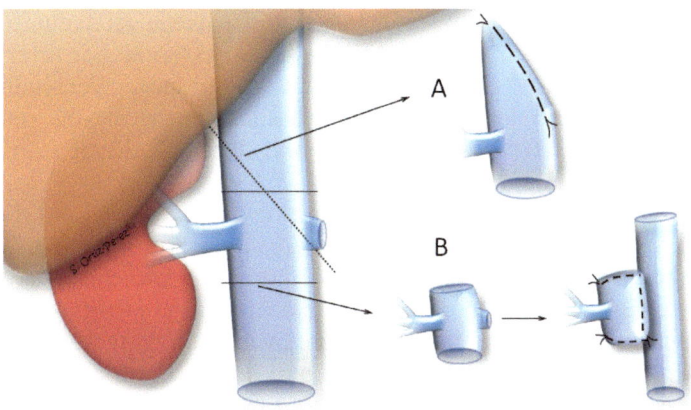

FIGURE 2.1 Venous extension of a right renal vein can be performed either with an oblique transection of the IVC (**A**) or side oversew of the supra- and infra-renal IVC ends (**B**). (*IVC* inferior vena cava, *RRV* right renal vein)

Initial sutures are placed either end of the venotomy with an anchor suture sometimes placed at the mid-point of the lateral wall to prevent the anterior or posterior wall being inadvertently caught up in the suture line. The anchoring sutures can prevent posterior wall suturing whilst ensuring end-to-side apposition.

Inaccessible or unsuitable iliac veins in the recipient can be managed by using the infrarenal and infra-hepatic inferior vena cava. In rare cases where both the iliac veins and the inferior vena cava have thrombosed, satisfactory results have been achieved with anastomosis of the renal vein to the portal venous drainage system, inferior and superior mesenteric veins and even large venous collaterals such as the left ovarian vein.

2.3.3.3   Arterial Anastomoses

Most operators would agree that surgical equipoise dictates personal preference over evidence base for the type of technique of renal artery to donor vessel anastomosis. Using a monofilament suture (5–0, 6–0 or 7–0), the most common vessel for end-to-side anastomosis is the external iliac artery (EIA), which is generally placed at a point more proximally than the vein, and for end-to-end anastomosis the internal iliac artery (IIA) in both living and deceased donor transplants remains the best option.

The external iliac artery is incised longitudinally and the lumen is irrigated with heparinized saline. An opening of a suitably-sized calibre created with an artery puncher is created in the common or external iliac artery and facilitates the anastomosis of renal arteries from live donors in the absence of Carrel patch. An endarterectomy is not needed in most cases, but if it is performed, any intimal flaps must be completely secured to the arterial wall with a tagging U-stitch. Taking full-thickness sutures of the arterial wall, particularly in patients with arteriosclerosis, must be meticulous to complete the anastomosis. The needle should move from inside to outside of the more diseased artery (usually the recipient artery) to tag the intima to the media of the artery and prevent creating of an intimal flap and potential thrombosis.

If a deceased donor graft has multiple vessels, a Carrel patch of aorta line with the graft vessels can be used. The patch technique, however, may result in elongated donor vessels (artery on the right side and vein on the left side) that leaves the graft vulnerable to kinking and could be a site of stenosis, thrombosis or drug-resistant hypertension at a later post-operative follow up. Dual arteries on a single patch to a right-sided kidney often make positioning of the kidney difficult without kinking one or the other artery, and might necessitate dividing the patch and shortening the arteries to fulfil two separate anastomoses. In addition, the Carrel patch may be severely atherosclerotic and might not be suitable for a safe anastomosis.

Multiple renal arteries in a living related donor represent more of a challenge. It is considered acceptable to ligate smaller arteries (less than 1 millimetre) of the upper and middle pole depending on the supply to the renal cortex. This can be judged during back-table perfusion of the kidney via the main donor vessel immediately after retrieval. Ligation is usually considered acceptable if the dependant area is judged to be less than 10%. Arteries bigger than 1 millimetre can be anastomosed to the EIA or possibly the inferior epigastric artery following reperfusion of the graft, especially in the lower pole to avoid ischaemia of the ureter. Smaller vessels (one to five millimetres) can be anastomosed using an interrupted monofilament (Prolene) suture that ensures an even distribution of tension around the vessel and prevents theoretical stricturing that can be caused with a continuous suture. In the living donor recipient setting, it is also the authors' experience to isolate a section of the distal IIA down towards the first branches and utilise the end for an end-to-end anastomosis with the main renal artery and then an end-to-side of the polar vessel directly onto the conduit (Fig. 2.2) or end-to-end with one of the first-order branches. Once the reconstruc-

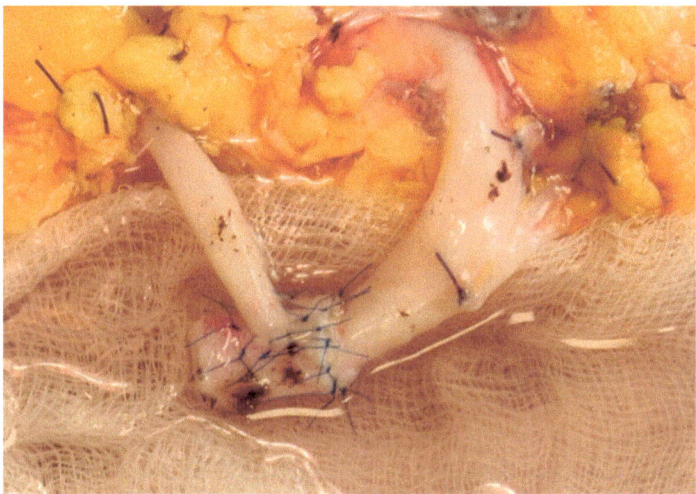

FIGURE 2.2 Use of the internal iliac artery conduit to create an end to end anastomosis of the main renal artery and end to side of the lower polar vessel. Interrupted 6–0 prolene sutures placed. (Picture courtesy of Mr. N Russell, Cambridge)

tion has been performed on the back table, the internal iliac end can be anastomosed back together with interrupted Prolene in an end-to-end fashion to the proximal IIA. The use of the internal iliac saves prolonged clamping of the EIA and leg ischaemia whilst preserving future options for the external iliac to be used.

Variant anatomy with two or more renal arteries may be anastomosed together side-to-side preserving the lumen of each vessel, or anastomosed separately to either the recipient EIA, IIA or one renal branch to each.

Different techniques may be employed if a surgeon attempts to reconstruct arteries before implantation including side-to-side anastomosis of same size arteries or end-to-side anastomosis of a smaller artery to a larger one (Fig. 2.3). In situations where the renal artery is damaged the best approach it is to transect the diseased part and use a small branch of the donor artery (for example, the donor iliac artery) as an elongation conduit of the renal artery. However, this would inevitably prolong the operative time and thus impact the length of warm ischaemia of the kidney.

2.3.3.4   Reperfusion

At the point of completion of the vascular anastomosis, vessel clamps can be removed to aid in reperfusion. It is the authors practise for reperfusion to coincide with a mean arterial pressure (MAP) of at least 65 mmHg with a systolic blood pressure of between 110 to 120 mmHg. At this point, the kidney is inspected for fullness of perfusion and then felt globally to ensure the organ is adequately filled. A soft kidney may be indicative of under filling or even arterial inflow problems, whereas an overly tense kidney could be a sign of venous outflow compromise. It is recommended that constant communication is held with the anaesthetist during the peri-reperfusion period so that changes in cardiovascular status is known and managed appropriately.

Potential challenges can occur with a non-perfused kidney and a pulsatile hilum- indicative of thrombosis or occlusion.

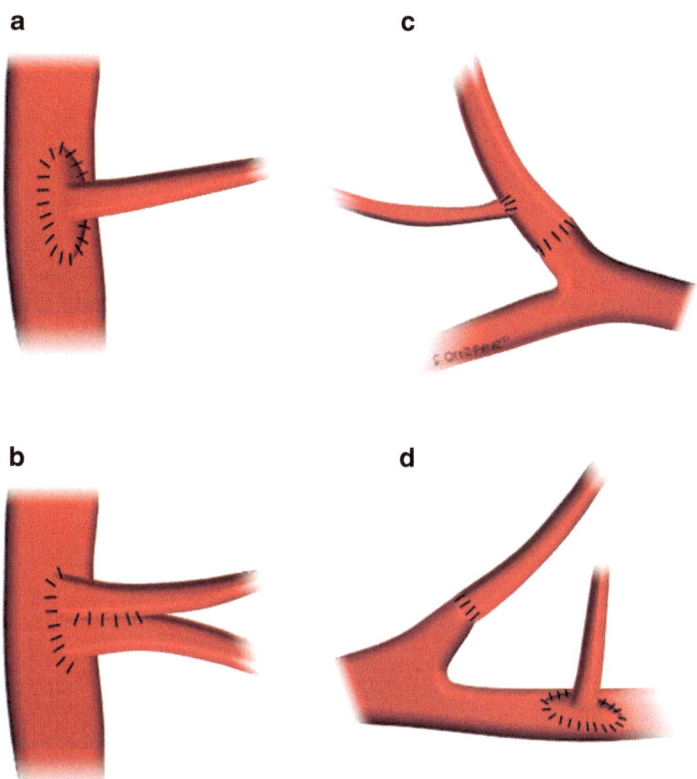

FIGURE 2.3 Some of the variant arterial anastomotic techniques. (a) standard end- to- side anastomosis with Carrel patch, (b) trouser side- to- side of 2 vessels with an end- to- side anastomosis to the external iliac artery, (c) end- to- end of the internal iliac with main artery and an end- to- side of the polar vessel to the artery, (d) use of the inferior epigastric artery for a lower polar artery

Intraoperative ultrasound can also be used to check flow within the artery and vein. At this point, preparation should be made to reclamp the iliac vessels, cold perfuse the organ with preservation solution and refashion the anastomoses. Preparation for blood loss should be made and it may be useful to consider cell salvage of blood.

2.3.3.5   Ureteric Implantation

The most common early post-operative complication in renal allograft transplantation (ranging from quoted rates of 5 to 10%) arises from the vesicoureteric anastomosis. Two major complications are recognised: urinary leak and ureteral stenosis. Prevention of these begins with meticulous attention to the surgical technique at time of implantation.

Urinary tract reconstruction begins following successful reperfusion of the donor kidney, with the type of reconstruction dependent on the position of the graft, condition of the recipient's bladder (or bladder alternative) and the length, condition and number of donor ureters. The most commonly employed technique is the ureteroneocystostomy (UNC) and is often categorised into transvesical or extravesical procedures. It is the authors' preference to keep the ureter as short as is feasible for a comfortable anastomosis to prevent distal ureteric ischaemia. Maintenance of the lower polar triangle of ureteric mesentery is essential given that blood supply to the upper ureter is originated from the lower polar terminal arterial branches.

The Leadbetter-Politano approach (transvesical UNC) utilises one anterior cystostomy to access the interior of the bladder and a posterior cystostomy to recreate a new ureteric orifice in the normal anatomical position, with the ureter subsequently tunnelled in the submucosa to prevent reflux. Murray et al. exploited this method during their first successful human renal transplant in 1954. The Lich-Gregoir technique (extravesical UNC) was first published in 1961, where the aim was to avoid a second cystostomy but maintain comparable antireflux mechanisms. The procedure consists of a suprahiatal detrusor myotomy and exposure of the bladder mucosa. Using either continuous or interrupted sutures the ureter is anastomosed to the mucosa with PDS II (polydioxanone) suture and then the detrusor muscle closed over it. Advantages compared to its counterpart procedure involve less bladder dissection, a shorter ureteral length and, overall, a quicker operative time associated with reduced morbidity.

A further variation of the extravesical approach to UNC includes the U-stitch technique, where after creating the anti-reflux tunnel (following dissection of the detrusor muscle and incision of the bladder mucosa), only one U-stitch at the toe or two U-stitches at the toe and the heel of the ureter are used to anchor it before closing with the detrusor muscle. This method can leave the anastomosis vulnerable to leakage, however, especially when there is concern about the distal ureteric blood supply and risk to ischaemia. Alternatively, two parallel incisions in the detrusor muscle may be used: one to transfer the ureter in a submucosal tunnel and the second to anastomose the ureter to the ureteral mucosa. Finally, the ureter may also be anastomosed to the full-thickness wall of the bladder without any antireflux mechanism.

Most surgeons use a ureteral stent to reduce the risk of obstruction in the post-operative period if the ureter or bladder tissue appears marginal. A meta-analysis evaluated five prospective, randomised, controlled trials of routine stenting vs no stenting following renal transplantation and indicated that the collective urinary complication rate following routine stenting was 1.5% compared to 9% without stenting. The markedly lowered incidence of ureteric complications, often a cause of graft loss, appeared to outweigh any increased risk of stent-associated problems such as urinary tract infections or bladder spasms. However, cystoscopic stent removal in the early period post transplantation (between 2 and 6 weeks) is imperative in order to avoid complications such as haematuria, stone formation and infection. Recent technological developments have enabled post-operative stent removal in the outpatient setting, with disposable instruments such as the Isiris™ (Coloplast, Humlebaek, Denmark) endoscope, complete with an incorporated camera module and grasper for the sole purpose of stent extraction. The solitary high cost of the single use camera is offset by the need of theatre space and a day surgery bed with conventional cystoscopy. Another innovation removes the need for cystoscopy altogether, with the ability to connect a magnet incorporated on the stent with that on the tip of a disposable catheter. The Magnetic Black Star retrieval catheter (Urotech, Achenmühle, Germany) is an introducer catheter smaller than a conventional urinary catheter and is designed for the sole purpose of retrieving the stent with the magnet in a single procedure. Unlike the Isiris system, no prior endoscopic experience is necessary and as such could be performed by a range of healthcare professionals.

In the case of a substandard graft ureter (too short, ischaemic or devascularised), or difficulty mobilising the bladder to enable a sufficient anastomosis, use of the native ureters may be necessary if there is clear lack of evidence for stricture, dilatation, reflux or infection. The surgeon may therefore perform an ureteroureterostomy, pyelouraterostomy or even pyeloneocystostomy. In rare cases where the renal transplant ureter and native ureter are both unsuitable, a pyelovesicostomy may be completed. Ureteral duplication is the most common congenital malformation of the urinary tract but there are few cases in the literature that describe renal transplantation with completely duplicated ureters. Bozkurt and colleagues used a modified extravesical UNC technique on a cadaveric kidney transplant with a completely duplicated ureter. The distal ends of the duplicated ureters were spatulated and their medial ends approximated before the distal parts were anastomosed to form a single cuff and subsequently sutured to the mucosa of the bladder. This approach differed to the previously described procedure involving anastomosis of both distal ends of the ureters to each other followed by the Lich-Gregoir technique for UNC.

2.3.3.6   Wound Closure

Given the potential morbidity associated with wound collections and dehiscence, judicious care should be taken when closing the kidney transplant wound. Mass closure can be adopted, although particular care must be taken in the upper lateral aspects of the external and internal oblique aponeurosis opposition to prevent incisional herniation or inadvertent bowel injury. A medium-sized silicon drain is commonly used which can be removed in the first few post operative days and this has the added advantage of reducing lymphatic collections immediately post operatively whilst being a safety measure for urinary leak should it occur.

2.3.3.7 Multiple Graft Implantation

In the current climate of growing transplant waiting lists and a shortage of organ donors, the use of extended criteria donors (ECD) is set to gain further momentum in the medium to short term. Extended criteria donors include donors aged 60 years and older or those aged over 50 years with at least two of the following three conditions: cerebrovascular cause of death, serum creatinine greater than 1.5 mg/ dL or a history of hypertension.

Outcomes of transplants from ECD kidneys are associated with higher rates of acute rejection episodes and long-term graft dysfunction. However, a benefit of extra life-years is still observed in recipients when compared to dialysis patients on the waiting list. Clinical characteristics that marginalise such donors include age, a history of hypertension or diabetes, the risk of transmitting infection or malignancy, brain death versus cardiac death, the presence of graft abnormalities as well as the morphology and functioning profile of the kidney.

One option for using organs from donors with a suboptimal nephron mass is dual kidney transplantation (DKT). This involves the simultaneous transplantation of two marginal kidneys from donors older than 60 years old or from a solitary paediatric patient younger than 5 years old or less than 21 kilograms in size. When retrieved from paediatric patients, the two kidneys are transplanted en-bloc and the aorta and inferior vena cava anastomosed to the external iliac artery and vein in an end-to-side technique.

Dual kidneys from older donors are mostly split for individual implantation either ipsilaterally or bilaterally in the iliac fossae of the recipient. Outcomes of dual kidneys from standard and extended criteria donors have been reported by a few centres. Remuzzi et al. outlined the use of a pathological scoring system in which risk was calculated based on histo-pathological analysis of the donor kidney biopsy. Grade of tubulitis, nephritis and vascular insult was stratified against outcome. This scoring system is now in use in some centres in the UK and a randomised national trial (PITHIA) of using this scoring sytem to allocate deceased donor kidneys (aged above 60 years) as single or duals is underway. With the availability of a 24 h pathology service that will risk stratify the quality of the donor kidney based on the Remuzzi score, it is predicted that each transplant unit's acceptance of kidneys for transplantation from elderly donors will increase by 10%.

A unilateral DKT is performed via a classic Gibson incision, preferably on the right side. The right kidney is placed superiorly as its renal vein may be lengthened by a segment of inferior vena cava. If necessary, the internal iliac vein can be divided to facilitate anastomosis of the renal vein to it and the renal artery anastomosed to the external iliac artery. Vascular clamps are placed immediately below the arterial and venous anastomoses following revascularisation of the right kidney; the left kidney is then implanted inferomedially and anastomosed also to the external iliac vessels. Extravesical ureteroneocystostomies are then performed separately leaving the ureter of the upper transplanted kidney lateral to the lower one.

2.3.4   Complications of Renal Transplantation

2.3.4.1   Wound Complications

Wound complications post kidney transplantation is by far the most common cause of morbidity with a reported incidence of around 5%. Risk factors associated with the development of wound issues can be categorised into patient related and drug related. Patient related factors include obesity, diabetes, clotting or pre-existing haematological disorders. The most common drug to cause wound problems in the early post-operative period is Sirolimus which has been associated with lymphocoele accumulation as well as dehiscence. Diagnosis is largely clinical, with local pain, erythema, discharge and dehiscence being common findings. Closure with skin clips enables local drainage of collections and the application of a superficial vacuum assisted closure (VAC) system. Treatment of wound infections with antibiotics should be guided based on positive microbiological cultures. Complete full thickness dehiscence of the wound is rare, but mandates return to theatre, wound washout and vacuum-assisted closure. Repeated exploration of patients for recurrent seromas or haematomas may give rise to the risk of incisional hernias which can be managed with mesh repair in the context of culture negative microbiology.

2.3.4.2   Arterial Complications

Post-transplantation transplant renal artery stenosis (TRAS) is not uncommon, with the varied reported rates of incidence of 0.5–13% in part attributed to lack of standardised definition of haemodynamically significant transplant renal artery stenosis. They can cause significant morbidity with transplant dysfunction and eventual graft failure.

The aetiology is complex with multiple predisposing factors such as pre-existing atherosclerosis, arterial trauma during transplant, cytomegalovirus infection and surgical technique. Transplant renal artery stenosis may arise in the donor renal artery, surgical anastomotic site or in the recipient iliac artery secondary to surgical trauma.

Initial evaluation of TRAS is most commonly performed by colour flow duplex ultrasound, with Magnetic resonance angiography (MRA) preserved for those with potentially complex vascular anatomy. Significant vascular stenosis is suggested by Doppler findings of: (i) peak systolic velocities >200 cm/second, (ii) velocity gradient between stenotic and prestenotic segment of >2:1, and (iii) distal turbulence seen as spectral broadening or parvus tardus waveform.

Institutions adopt varying intervention management strategies, with some performing percutaneous angioplasty (PTA) and solely reserving stents for balloon-resistant stenoses as the primary percutaneous intervention. Primary angioplasty is often implemented in those with stenosis affecting the mainstem or first-order segmental arteries, whilst stent placement is performed in case of residual stenosis or dissection.

A meta-analysis reported a higher technical success (98% vs 77%), lower restenosis rate (17% vs 26%) and clinical outcome (20% vs 10% cure rate in hypertension, and 30 vs 38% improvement rate of renal function, $p < 0.001$) in stent placement compared to angioplasty alone.

Conservative management of TRAS has a higher risk of graft failure (65%) with early intervention. Medical management is advocated if the stenosis is considered haemodynamically insignificant or if intervention is deemed to be associated with high risk of graft loss. In a retrospective single centre study of 44 primary angioplasty treated TRAS, 82% demonstrated improvement in graft function, with this cohort being the only one illustrating both significant and sustained improvement in BP blood pressure and serum creatinine, compared to groups treated with surgery or conservative medical management. Surgery is reserved for those refractory or with unfavourable anatomy for PTA. Other indications for surgery include recent transplant, multiple stenoses, long and narrow stenoses.

2.3.4.3   Venous Complications

Venous thrombosis is relatively rare but a clinically devastating post-operative complication (2.9% in one study of 103 renal transplants (41), with rates ranging from 0.5% to 4%. It should be considered in the presence of acute severe suprapubic swelling or sudden onset frank haematuria and is most common within the first 30 days post-operatively. Even though there are many intrinsic causes of thrombosis, it is more likely that in the immediate post-operative setting the cause is due to kinking of the renal vein or the onset of sustained hypotension. Of note, numerous retrospective studies have found that intraoperative heparin did not reduce the incidence of graft thrombosis. Despite some solitary case reports of thrombolysis, the usual treatment of choice is graft salvage with a reoperation and thrombectomy and most likely graft nephrectomy. The choice of anticoagulation post -operatively will be balanced against the risk of bleeding or collections, but it is the authors experience that haematomas and collections are easier to manage than thrombotic episodes.

2.3.4.4   Ureteric Complications

Despite the widespread use of intraoperative placement of transplant ureteric stents, the reported ureteric complication rate is widely quoted from 2–4%. Ureteric complications are largely leak related or obstructive (stenosis or external compression from, for example, a lymphocoele). Clinical evidence of a leak can be in the form of suprapubic or graft site tenderness in the setting of oliguria or with a differentially high drain creatinine. The cause of this in the immediate post operative setting is either technical or necrosis due to an ischaemic ureter. Management of leaks is almost always drainage of the collection followed by surgical correction, although temporising ureteric stents can be placed in the context of minor leaks.

A longer term complication in the setting of insidious graft dysfunction and sonographic features of hydronephrosis, is ureteric stenosis. This can occur over several weeks to months and can be associated with infection (e.g. BK virus), ischaemia or rejection. Initial management must confirm the absence of infection, temporising urinary drainage with a percutaneous nephrostomy prior to definitive treatment. This is then followed with either balloon ureteroplasty for short segment stenosis or surgical reimplantation of a healthy section of the donor ureter. The latter can be performed directly back on to the bladder itself or implanting the native ureter onto the transplant pelvic ureteric junction in the case of lengthy stenotic lesions.

2.3.4.5   Lymphocoele Formation

The disruption of lymphatics either during dissection of the iliac vasculature in the recipient or during procurement of the kidney and preparation of the renal hilum, can cause collections of lymph post-operatively. Documented incidence of lymphocoeles range from 0.6 to 18% making it one of the most common causes of early morbidity in the renal transplant recipient. Diagnosis is based on graft dysfunction with the presence of a collection surrounding classically the lower pole of the kidney on sonography. Aspiration of the collection can confirm the lymphocoele, rather than a urinoma, when sent for biochemistry and measurment of creatinine. Management can be either percutaneous or open drainage, with fenestration of the peritoneum under open or laparoscopic vision. This should be performed with judicious balance towards drainage of the lymph in a sizeable window without risking the development of intestinal herniation. Excellent results have been seen with laparoscopic approaches to lymph drainage compared to open. Another option is the injection of a sclerosant such as iodine, tetracycline or fibrin glue, although mixed outcomes in terms of rates of complete resolution have been reported.

2.4   Future Perspectives

Kidney transplantation has become the optimal treatment for patients with end-stage renal disease. Early recognition and management of post-operative complications is key to minimising patient morbidity, and potentially mortality, attributed to graft loss. Variation in surgical implantation site has evolved with the advent of multivisceral procedures and the inclusion of suboptimal grafts. Thoughtful consideration must be given to the use of kidneys from extended criteria donors (ECD) and the implementation of dual kidney transplantation (DKT) which can be associated with a higher risk of surgical complications when compared to a standard kidney transplant. Finally, a consensus is required regarding intraoperative or post-operative anticoagulation avoid peri- or post-operative graft thrombosis as recent evidence suggests little to no benefit over no anticoagulation.

Of course, not to be overlooked is the development, advancement and clinical integration of robotic technology in renal transplant surgery. The first case report of laparoscopic/robotic kidney transplantation was published in 2010 demonstrating the feasibility of such a procedure; however, operative anastomosis time was slower when compared in other studies with open kidney transplantation. Nevertheless, limited published data report less pain, better cosmetic appearance, fewer wound complications resulting in shorter hospital stay, and equivocal graft function to an open procedure. It is clear that with refinement of laparoscopic devices and technique, this is a strategy that may be widely employed in the near future. The current limitation of high cost with an equivocal outcome measure over conventional open implantation means uptake is likely to be slow, with significant benefits potentially to be seen in sub-group of patients e.g. those with high BMI.

Finally, perfusion machine systems have been one of the most exciting developments in the last decade. The initial cold perfusion machine of the Lifeport™ (Organ Recovery Systems,Brussels, Belgium) that was trialled across the UK and Europe, has been shown to reduce the incidence of delayed graft function and lead to better graft function at 3 years in a recent meta-analysis. More recently, ex-vivo normothermic perfusion (EVNP) of kidneys has been developed by by Hosgood and associates and offers the potential to serve as a tool for evaluation of kidney grafts prior to implanatation in order to reduce the uncertainty with respect to graft viability often encountered when using marginal kidneys. This has led to a multi-centre clinical trial aimed at establishing whether EVNP can improve early graft function in DCD kidney transplants.

Finally, whilst at the experimental phase, the potential for establishing cellular treatments or repair using the machine perfusion platform, for example by infusion of nanoparticles attached with therapeutic drugs directly into the donor kidney, remains an exciting prospect.

Bibliography

1. Klein AA, Lewis CJ, Madsen JC. Organ transplantation; a clinical guide: Cambridge University Press; 2011.
2. Libby P, Pober JS. Chronic rejection. Immunity. 2001;14(4):387–97.
3. Pascual M, Theruvath T, Kawai T, Tolkoff-Rubin N, Cosimi AB. Strategies to improve long-term outcomes after renal transplantation. N Engl J Med. 2002;346(8):580–90.
4. Heaphy EL, Poggio ED, Flechner SM, Goldfarb DA, Askar M, Fatica R, et al. Risk factors for retransplant kidney recipients: relisting and outcomes from patients' primary transplant. Am J Transplant. 2014;14(6):1356–67.
5. Nankivell BJ, Borrows RJ, Fung CL, O'Connell PJ, Allen RD, Chapman JR. The natural history of chronic allograft nephropathy. N Engl J Med. 2003;349(24):2326–33.
6. Muzaale AD, Massie AB, Wang MC, Montgomery RA, McBride MA, Wainright JL, et al. Risk of end-stage renal disease following live kidney donation. JAMA. 2014;311(6):579–86.
7. Mjoen G, Hallan S, Hartmann A, Foss A, Midtvedt K, Oyen O, et al. Long-term risks for kidney donors. Kidney Int. 2014;86(1):162–7.
8. Matas AJ, Wadstrom J, Ibrahim HN. Kidney donation and risk of ESRD. JAMA. 2014;312(1):92–3.
9. Heimbach JK, Taler SJ, Prieto M, Cosio FG, Textor SC, Kudva YC, et al. Obesity in living kidney donors: clinical characteristics and outcomes in the era of laparoscopic donor nephrectomy. Am J Transplant. 2005;5(5):1057–64.
10. Kalantar-Zadeh K, Kopple JD. Body mass index and risk for end-stage renal disease. Ann Intern Med. 2006;144(9):701; author reply 701–2.
11. Vivante A, Golan E, Tzur D, Leiba A, Tirosh A, Skorecki K, et al. Body mass index in 1.2 million adolescents and risk for end-stage renal disease. Arch Intern Med. 2012;172(21):1644–50.

12. Yang A, Barman N, Chin E, Herron D, Arvelakis A, LaPointe Rudow D, et al. Robotic-assisted vs. laparoscopic donor nephrectomy: a retrospective comparison of perioperative course and postoperative outcome after 1 year. J Robot Surg. 2018;12(2):343–50.
13. Minnee RC, Bemelman WA, Maartense S, Bemelman FJ, Gouma DJ, Idu MM. Left or right kidney in hand-assisted donor nephrectomy? A randomized controlled trial. Transplantation. 2008;85(2):203–8.
14. Hsu TH, Su L, Ratner LE, Trock BJ, Kavoussi LR. Impact of renal artery multiplicity on outcomes of renal donors and recipients in laparoscopic donor nephrectomy. Urology. 2003;61(2):323–7.
15. Saidi R, Kawai T, Kennealey P, Tsouflas G, Elias N, Hertl M, et al. Living donor kidney transplantation with multiple arteries: recent increase in modern era of laparoscopic donor nephrectomy. Arch Surg. 2009;144(5):472–5.
16. Gerstenkorn C, Papalois VE, Thomusch O, Maxwell AP, Hakim N. Surgical management of multiple donor veins in renal transplantation. Int Surg. 2006;91(6):345–7.
17. Tran MH, Foster CE, Kalantar-Zadeh K, Ichii H. Kidney transplantation in obese patients. World J Transplant. 2016;6(1):135–43.
18. Rahul Koushik BK. Chapter 16: kidney transplantation-the recipient: Mc Graw Hill Medical; 2008.
19. Ratner LE, Ciseck LJ, Moore RG, Cigarroa FG, Kaufman HS, Kavoussi LR. Laparoscopic live donor nephrectomy. Transplantation. 1995;60(9):1047–9.
20. Giessing M. Laparoscopic living-donor nephrectomy. Nephrology Dialysis Transplant 2004;19:36–40.
21. Kokkinos C, Nanidis T, Antcliffe D, Darzi AW, Tekkis P, Papalois V. Comparison of laparoscopic versus hand-assisted live donor nephrectomy. Transplantation. 2007;83(1):41–7.
22. Nanidis TG, Antcliffe D, Kokkinos C, Borysiewicz CA, Darzi AW, Tekkis PP, et al. Laparoscopic versus open live donor nephrectomy in renal transplantation: a meta-analysis. Ann Surg. 2008;247(1):58–70.
23. Horgan S, Vanuno D, Sileri P, Cicalese L, Benedetti E. Robotic-assisted laparoscopic donor nephrectomy for kidney transplantation. Transplantation. 2002;73(9):1474–9.
24. Giacomoni A, Di Sandro S, Lauterio A, Concone G, Buscemi V, Rossetti O, et al. Robotic nephrectomy for living donation:

surgical technique and literature systematic review. Am J Surg. 2016;211(6):1135–42.

25. Segev DL, Muzaale AD, Caffo BS, Mehta SH, Singer AL, Taranto SE, et al. Perioperative mortality and long-term survival following live kidney donation. JAMA. 2010;303(10):959–66.

26. Patel S, Cassuto J, Orloff M, Tsoulfas G, Zand M, Kashyap R, et al. Minimizing morbidity of organ donation: analysis of factors for perioperative complications after living-donor nephrectomy in the United States. Transplantation. 2008;85(4):561–5.

27. Mjoen G, Oyen O, Holdaas H, Midtvedt K, Line PD. Morbidity and mortality in 1022 consecutive living donor nephrecto- mies: benefits of a living donor registry. Transplantation. 2009;88(11):1273–9.

28. Hadjianastassiou VG, Johnson RJ, Rudge CJ, Mamode N. 2509 living donor nephrectomies, morbidity and mortality, includ- ing the UK introduction of laparoscopic donor surgery. Am J Transplant. 2007;7(11):2532–7.

29. Ibrahim HN, Foley R, Tan L, Rogers T, Bailey RF, Guo H, et al. Long-term consequences of kidney donation. N Engl J Med. 2009;360(5):459–69.

30. Clemens KK, Thiessen-Philbrook H, Parikh CR, Yang RC, Karley ML, Boudville N, et al. Psychosocial health of living kidney donors: a systematic review. Am J Transplant. 2006;6(12):2965–77.

31. Smith GC, Trauer T, Kerr PG, Chadban SJ. Prospective psy- chosocial monitoring of living kidney donors using the short Form-36 health survey: results at 12 months. Transplantation. 2004;78(9):1384–9.

32. Andersen MH, Mathisen L, Veenstra M, Oyen O, Edwin B, Digernes R, et al. Quality of life after randomization to laparo- scopic versus open living donor nephrectomy: long-term follow- up. Transplantation. 2007;84(1):64–9.

33. Perry KT, Freedland SJ, Hu JC, Phelan MW, Kristo B, Gritsch AH, et al. Quality of life, pain and return to normal activities following laparoscopic donor nephrectomy versus open mini- incision donor nephrectomy. J Urol. 2003;169(6):2018–21.

34. Buell JF, Lee L, Martin JE, Dake NA, Cavanaugh TM, Hanaway MJ, et al. Laparoscopic donor nephrectomy vs. open live donor nephrectomy: a quality of life and functional study. Clin Transpl. 2005;19(1):102–9.

35. Nicholson ML, Elwell R, Kaushik M, Bagul A, Hosgood SA. Health-related quality of life after living donor nephrectomy: a randomized controlled trial of laparoscopic versus open nephrectomy. Transplantation. 2011;91(4):457–61.

36. Morris PJ. Transplantation–a medical miracle of the 20th century. N Engl J Med. 2004;23(351(26)):2.

37. Cassini MF, de Andrade MF, Tucci S. Surgical Complications of Renal Transplantation.

38. Gittes RF, Waters WB. Sexual impotence: the overlooked complication of a second renal transplant. J Urol. 1979;121(6):719–20.

39. Nanni G, Tondolo V, Citterio F, Romagnoli J, Borgetti M, Boldrini G, et al. Comparison of oblique versus hockey-stick surgical incision for kidney transplantation. Transplant Proc. 2005;37(6):2479–81.

40. Khan T. Post kidney transplant lymphoceles: meticulous ligation of lymphatics reduces incidence. 2011.

41. Baston CHM, Preda A, Gener I, Manea I, Voinea S, et al. Comparative urologic complications of ureteroneocystostomy in kidney transplantation: transvesical Leadbetter-Politano versus extravesical lich-Gregoir technique. Transplant Proc. 2014;46(1):3.

42. Zilinska ZCM, Trebaticky B, Breza J, Slobodnik L, Breza J, et al. Vascular complications after renal transplantation. Bratisl Lekárske Listy. 2010;111(11):3.

43. Mangus RSHB. Stented versus nonstented extravesical ureteroneocystostomy in renal transplantation: a metaanalysis. Am J Transplant. 2004;4(11):7.

44. MT. BB. Modified extravesical ureteroneocystostomy in cadaveric kidney transplantation with completely duplicated ureters: a case report. J Transplant Technol Res. 2014;04(2).

45. NHSBT. Taking organ transplantation to 2020. In: England N, editor. Bristol: NHSBT; 2018.

46. Aubert O, Kamar N, Vernerey D, Viglietti D, Martinez F, Duong-Van-Huyen JP, et al. Long term outcomes of transplantation using kidneys from expanded criteria donors: prospective, population based cohort study. BMJ. 2015;351:h3557.

47. Lucarelli G, Bettocchi C, Battaglia M, Impedovo SV, Vavallo A, Grandaliano G, et al. Extended criteria donor kidney transplantation: comparative outcome analysis between single ver-

sus double kidney transplantation at 5 years. Transplant Proc. 2010;42(4):1104–7.

48. Remuzzi G, Grinyo J, Ruggenenti P, Beatini M, Cole EH, Milford EL, et al. Early experience with dual kidney transplantation in adults using expanded donor criteria. Double kidney transplant group (DKG). J Am Soc Nephrol. 1999;10(12):2591–8.

49. Remuzzi G, Ruggenenti P. Renal transplantation: single or dual for donors aging > or =60 years? Transplantation. 2000;69(10):2000–1.

50. Schaffer M, Schier R, Napirei M, Michalski S, Traska T, Viebahn R. Sirolimus impairs wound healing. Langenbeck's Arch Surg. 2007;392(3):297–303.

51. Kobayashi KCM, Rossman LL, Kyriakides PN, Kahan BD, Cohen AM. Interventional radiologic management of renal transplant dysfunction: indications, limitations, and technical considerations. Radiographics. 2007;27(4).

52. Ghazanfar ATA, Augustine T, Pararajasingam R, Riad H, Chalmers N. Management of transplant renal artery stenosis and its impact on long-term allograft survival: a single-Centre experience. Nephrol Dial Transplant. 2011;26(1):7.

53. Voiculescu ASM, Hollenbeck M, Braasch S, Luther B, Sandmann W, Jung G, Mödder U, Grabensee B. Management of arterial stenosis affecting kidney graft perfusion: a single-centre study in 53 patients. Am J Transplant. 2005;5(7):7.

54. Leertouwer TCGE, Bosch JL, van Jaarsveld BC, van Dijk LC, Deinum J, Man In 't Veld AJ. Stent placement for renal arterial stenosis: where do we stand? A meta-analysis. Radiology. 2000;216(1):7.

55. Baig MA, Khan T, Mousa D. Post transplant ureteric stenosis causing allograft hydronephrosis and calyceal rupture: salvage side to side ureteroneocystostomy. Saudi J Kidney Dis Transpl. 2010;21(3):504–6.

56. Keller H, Noldge G, Wilms H, Kirste G. Incidence, diagnosis, and treatment of ureteric stenosis in 1298 renal transplant patients. Transpl Int. 1994;7(4):253–7.

57. Golriz M, Klauss M, Zeier M, Mehrabi A. Prevention and management of lymphocele formation following kidney transplantation. Transplant Rev (Orlando). 2017;31(2):100–5.

58. Lucewicz A, Wong G, Lam VW, Hawthorne WJ, Allen R, Craig JC, et al. Management of primary symptomatic lymphocele after

kidney transplantation: a systematic review. Transplantation. 2011;92(6):663–73.

59. Wagenaar S, Nederhoed JH, Hoksbergen AWJ, Bonjer HJ, Wisselink W, van Ramshorst GH. Minimally invasive, laparoscopic, and robotic-assisted techniques versus open techniques for kidney transplant recipients: a systematic review. Eur Urol. 2017;72(2):205–17.

60. Hosgood SA, Yang B, Bagul A, Mohamed IH, Nicholson ML. A comparison of hypothermic machine perfusion versus static cold storage in an experimental model of renal ischemia reperfusion injury. Transplantation. 2010;89(7):830–7.

61. Jochmans I, O'Callaghan JM, Pirenne J, Ploeg RJ. Hypothermic machine perfusion of kidneys retrieved from standard and high-risk donors. Transplant international: official journal of the European society for. Organ Transplantation. 2015;28(6):665–76.

62. Hosgood SA, Barlow AD, Hunter JP, Nicholson ML. Ex vivo normothermic perfusion for quality assessment of marginal donor kidney transplants. Br J Surg. 2015;102(11):1433–40.

63. Chadha R, Hossain MA, Bagul A. Optimising organs for transplantation: is normothermic machine perfusion the answer? Expert Rev Med Devices. 2016;13(3):221–3.

64. Doizi S, Kamphuis G, Giusti G, Palmero JL, Patterson JM, Proietti S, Straub M, De La Rosette J, Traxer O. First clinical evaluation of a new single-use flexible cystoscope dedicated to double-J stent removal (Isiris™): a European prospective multicenter study. World J Urol. 2017;35(8):1269–75.

65. Rassweiler MC, Michel MS, Ritter M, Honeck P. Magnetic ureteral stent removal without cystoscopy: a randomized controlled trial. J Endourol. 2017;31(8):762–6.

66. Mallon DH, Riddiough GE, Summers DM, Butler AJ, Callaghan CJ, Bradbury LL, Bardsley V, Broecker V, Saeb-Parsy K, Torpey N, Bradley JA, Pettigrew GJ. Successful transplantation of kidneys from elderly circulatory death donors by using microscopic and macroscopic characteristics to guide single or dual implantation. Am J Transplant. 2015;15(11):2931–9.

67. Ekser B, Furian L, Broggiato A, Silvestre C, Pierobon ES, Baldan N, Rigotti P. Technical aspects of unilateral dual kidney transplantation from expanded criteria donors: experience of 100 patients. Am J Transplant. 2010;10(9):2000–7.

68. Ayorinde JO, Summers DM, Pankhurst L, Laing E, Deary AJ, Hemming K, Wilson ECF, Bardsley V, Neil DA, Pettigrew GJ. PreImplantation Trial of Histopathology In renal Allografts (PITHIA): a stepped-wedge cluster randomised controlled trial protocol. BMJ Open. 2019;9(1):e026166.

69. Snanoudj R, Timsit MO, Rabant M, Tinel C, Lazareth H, Lamhaut L, Martinez F, Legendre C. Dual kidney transplantation: is it worth it? Transplantation. 2017;101(3):488–97.

70. van den Berg TAJ, Minnee RC, Nieuwenhuijs-Moeke GJ, Bakker SJL, Pol RA. The effect of perioperative antiplatelet/ anticoagulant therapy on the incidence of early postoperative thromboembolic complications and bleeding in kidney transplantation. - a dual center retrospective cohort study of 2000 kidney transplant recipients. Transplantation. 2018;102:S186.

71. Eng M, Brock G, Li X, Chen Y, Ravindra KV, Buell JF, Marvin MR. Perioperative anticoagulation and antiplatelet therapy in renal transplant: is there an increase in bleeding complication? Clin Transpl. 2011;25(2):292–6.

72. Breda A, Territo A, Gausa L, Tuğcu V, Alcaraz A, Musquera M, Decaestecker K, Desender L, Stockle M, Janssen M, Fornara P, Mohammed N, Siena G, Serni S, Guirado L, Facundo C, Doumerc N. Robot-assisted kidney transplantation: the European experience. Eur Urol. 2018;73(2):273–81.

73. Sood A, Ghosh P, Menon M, Jeong W, Bhandari M, Ahlawat R. Robotic renal transplantation: current status. J Minim Access Surg. 2015;11(1):35.

74. Peng P, Ding Z, He Y, Zhang J, Wang X, Yang Z. Hypothermic machine perfusion versus static cold storage in deceased donor kidney transplantation: a systematic review and meta-analysis of randomized controlled trials. Artif Organs. 2018;43(5):478–89.

75. Hosgood SA, Saeb-Parsy K, Wilson C, Callaghan C, Collett D, Nicholson ML. Protocol of a randomised controlled, open-label trial of ex vivo normothermic perfusion versus static cold storage in donation after circulatory death renal transplantation. BMJ Open. 2017;7(1):e012237.

76. Bahmani B, Uehara M, Jiang L, Ordikhani F, Banouni N, Ichimura T, Solhjou Z, Furtmüller GJ, Brandacher G, Alvarez D, von Andrian UH, Uchimura K, Xu Q, Vohra I, Yilmam OA, Haik Y, Azzi J, Kasinath V, Bromberg JS, McGrath MM,

Abdi R. Targeted delivery of immune therapeutics to lymph nodes prolongs cardiac allograft survival. J Clin Investig. 2018;128(11):4770–86.

77. Hosgood SA, Thompson E, Moore T, Wilson CH, Nicholson ML. Normothermic machine perfusion for the assessment and transplantation of declined human kidneys from donation after circulatory death donors. Br J Surg. 2018;105(4):388–94.

Chapter 3
Pancreas Transplantation

Gabriele Spoletini and Steven A. White

3.1   Introduction

A functioning pancreatic allograft is the sole long-term
option to maintain euglycemia in insulin-dependent patients
without exposing them to the risks of severe hypoglycemia.
The transplant provides the chance of halting the progression of chronic diabetic complications and in some situations
reversing them.

Diabetes mellitus (DM) with its complications is a pan-
demic disease causing a significant healthcare burden.
Worldwide, 425 million people have DM and over a million
children and adolescents have type 1 DM. Acute complications include life threatening ketoacidosis and hyperosmotic
coma for type 1 and type 2 diabetes (T1DM and T2DM),
respectively. Chronic exposure to elevated blood glucose
leads to micro and macrovascular changes affecting most
organs such as heart and cerebrovascular disease, renal failure, blindness and limb amputation.

Conventional insulin therapy is effective in limiting the
acute metabolic effects of hyperglycemia, while its impact

G. Spoletini (✉) · S. A. White
Transplant Surgery Unit, Freeman Hospital, Newcastle
Upon Tyne Hospitals, Newcastle, UK
e-mail: Gabriele.spoletini@nhs.net

© Springer Nature Switzerland AG 2019   119
R. Díaz-Nieto (ed.), *Procurement and Transplantation of
Abdominal Organs in Clinical Practice*, In Clinical Practice,
https://doi.org/10.1007/978-3-030-21370-1_3

on diabetic comorbidities is less profound, as shown in the Diabetes Control and Complications Trial and Epidemiology of Diabetes Interventions and Complications trial, revealing that intensive glucose control can mitigate some microvascular complications, though the risk of potentially life-threatening insulin-induced hypoglycemia persists. The annual mortality rate of patients with insulin-induced inadvertent hypoglycemia is estimated to be as high as 3–6%.

Current treatment options for diabetes are aimed at eliminating symptoms due to acute metabolic imbalance, preventing the development of chronic complications of the disease and extending and improving the quality of life. Glycemic control is the main focus of treatment, and glycosylated hemoglobin (HbA1c) is the most common parameter to monitor diabetes control. Maintaining HbA1c levels to <7% has shown to be effective for the prevention of the development of chronic complications related to the disease. The target may be decreased further (e.g. to 6.0% – 6.5%) in patients with long life expectancy provided this does not increase the frequency of episodes of hypoglycemia. Conversely, in patients with a shorter life expectancy, with already significant micro and macrovascular disease or in those at higher risk of hypoglycemia, HbA1c levels may be set above 7%.

Among treatment options, lifestyle interventions focused on dietary changes, increased physical activity and weight loss when needed, are fundamental components in the management of diabetes.

The mainstay of treatment in type 1 diabetes is exogenous insulin injections. Since the discovery of insulin, there have been great endeavors to try replicate its endogenous pharmacokinetics and pharmacodynamics. A number of types insulins and analogues are available, and routes of administrations vary too. From standard subcutaneous injections to continuous infusion and more recently closed loop infusion. Despite intensified insulin regimens improving HbA1c levels and reducing the rate of long-term complications, it does not prevent them. Also, wide fluctuations in glucose levels and the

risk of hypoglycemic episodes - specifically in patients with
T1DM - remain common. Because there is no system available yet to replicate the continuous physiological adjustment
of insulin secretion, the only way to achieve fully regulated
normoglycemia is beta cell replacement therapy. (However in
recent years, refinements in insulin pumps and the addition
of glucose sensors have proven effective in reducing HbA1c
levels without increasing the risk of hypoglycemia.

In 20 to 30% of patients with type 2 diabetes, exogenous
insulin administration is required. This latter group of patients
typically receive treatment with oral agents and non-insulin
injectable drugs. However, patients with T2DM with poor
glycemic regulation suffer the same life-threatening complications as in T1DM, such as severe hypoglycemia and uremia.
Over the last few years, the number of SPK in patients with
T2DM has steadily increased but the rate of solitary pancreas
transplants still remains low.

3.2   Indications for Pancreas Transplantation

Pancreas transplantation (PTX) is aimed at providing a functioning beta-cell mass with the effect of restoring euglycemia
in patients with diabetes. Those who benefit the most from
PTX are those with complicated diabetes, in whom the risks
of surgery and immunosuppression are deemed to be lower
than those having ineffective conventional insulin therapy.
When diabetic nephropathy is also present, a kidney transplant should be added.

Since the first case in 1966, PTX has become a safe and
effective therapy for type 1 diabetes and a potential treatment
modality in selected cases of type 2 diabetes. Still, due to its
relatively high morbidity, patients are eligible for a pancreas
transplant only if they have or are at high risk of secondary
complications of diabetes, have disabling or life-threatening
hypoglycemic unawareness, or are likely to develop these and
are deemed fit enough to survive the operation.

Depending on patient co-morbidity (fitness for surgery), renal function, and availability of a living donor, there are three main modalities of PTX:

1. Pancreas transplant alone (PTA): for patients with T1DM with frequent and severe episodes of hypoglycemia and/or unawareness, impaired quality of life, issues related to noncompliance with insulin therapy and preserved renal function. Around 30% of those receiving a PTA will eventually need a kidney transplant 9 or 10 years later because of the detrimental cumulative effects of immunosuppression with calcineurin inhibitors. Patients with a GFR of less than 80 mL/min at the time of PTA, are more likely to require a kidney transplant than those with higher baseline kidney function. In addition, after a PTA there is a more rapid deterioration in GFR than with intensified insulin regimen. However, the worsening of interstitial fibrosis and tubular atrophy observed at 5 years post-PTA, consequent to cyclosporine therapy can improve 10 years after PTA.

2. Simultaneous pancreas kidney transplant (SPK) is indicated in type 1 diabetics with end stage renal failure requiring immediate dialysis or within 6 months. However, some patients can be pre-emptively transplanted before loss of kidney function reaches the window of 6 months (e.g. in the UK once GFR falls below 20 ml/min/1.73m^2). Recipients of a pre-emptive SPK have better survival 8 years after transplantation when compared with those transplanted while already on dialysis. The main advantage of SPK is the increased rate of success of the pancreas graft because concurrent acute rejection in both organs can be recognized by an increase in serum creatinine concentrations. Also, a synergistic protective effect is exerted by the kidney when transplanted together with other organs from the same donor, the mechanism of which is not entirely clarified. SPK improves patient survival compared to dialysis treatment or deceased donor kidney transplantation (KTX) alone. Patients survival while on the waiting list for a SPK were of 93.4% and 58.7% compared to post-SPK survival

rates of 95.0% and 90.3% respectively, as reported by the University of Minnesota

3. Pancreas after kidney (PAK): for post-uremic patients (i.e. those who have already undergone either a living or deceased donor KTX), is aimed at protecting the transplanted kidney from the detrimental effects of diabetes. The benefits include a shorter waiting time and reduced mortality rate when compared to SPK patients (because of the correction of uremia, also the reduced complexity of the operation), and a reduction in time on dialysis especially for those who receive a living donor kidney transplant: this approach supposedly outweighs the immunologic advantage of an SPK transplant and also by adding the longevity of a living donor kidney (i.e. two organs from different donors instead of two organs from the same donor) (.

Living donor segmental pancreas transplants (LDSPTX) have been performed selectively to offer a preemptive transplant option for SPK recipients and to perform a single operation decreasing the cost of PAK transplant. This option historically provided a better immunologic match (thanks to living-related donation). The immunologic advantages are emphasized in highly sensitized recipients of PTA who, with cadaver donation, wait the longest time and face the poorest outcome. Furthermore, LD allows recipient pre-conditioning and/or pair donor exchange. However, morbidity risk and the onset of DM in the donor (10–20%) are consistent and led to criticism. LDSPTX may play an important role in countries where organ donation from deceased donors is less widespread (i.e. Eastern countries) and in highly selected recipients with little options for cadaveric donation.

Alternatively to solid organ PTX, improved results compared to the past are now achieved with islet transplantation (ITX), especially since the introduction of the glucocorticoid-free 'Edmonton' immunosuppressive protocol in 2000. ITX can be combined with KTX in various modalities to the point of some centers now offering islets after or simultaneously to kidney transplantation (respectively IAK and SIK). Preferentially, ITX is recommended in patients with higher surgical risk for solid organ transplantation, mainly due to diabetes-related comorbidities, and of older age or patient preference.

Solid organ transplantation is preferable in younger candidates, where a longer insulin independence is auspicated, with larger body habitus and higher insulin requirements. Ideally islet transplant alone should be limited to patients who necessitate up to 43 units of insulin per day or 0.6 units/kg. The increased morbidity and mortality risk with PTX is counterbalanced by the more durable effect, whereas with ITX it is accepted that repeated islets infusions will be required in the future, mainly due to a progressive burn out of the beta cells. Also, because the yield of viable islets from a single pancreas is inferior to those present within a whole transplanted pancreas, in most cases more than one organ is needed to provide the recipient with a functioning islet transplant. This makes ITX a less efficient resource than PTX. Another difference between ITX and PTX is that the primary goal of current ITX is not insulin independence (as is the case with pancreas transplants) but rather a reduction in the incidence and severity of hypoglycemic events, a reduction in exogenous insulin requirements, an increase in measurable C-peptide levels and an amelioration of HbA1c levels.

3.3   Pancreas Donation and Allocation

Overall, in the last decade there has been a decrease in the activity of PTX worldwide, particularly in US centers. (Mainly, changing demographics (older and more obese donors and recipients), improved pharmacological diabetes control and glucose sensors, improvements in islet transplantation and the general perception of the morbidity and mortality risk associated to PTX, are all responsible for such a decrease. Especially in the UK and a few other countries, this phenomenon has been partly counterbalanced by an overall increase in the number of donor organs such as donors after circulatory death (DCD) along with a higher usage of more marginal donors (i.e. higher BMI, age and/or DCD) has been instrumental to maintain the volumes of work in many transplant centers.

Strict selection criteria are adopted by most centers, mainly because PTX is not an immediate life-saving procedure rather life improving and the risk of peri-operative complications (including life-threatening) is increased when utilizing pancreas grafts from more marginal donors. After the enthusiasm in the early millennium years and broadening of donor criteria, the subsequent higher rates of technical complications (i.e. thrombosis and graft pancreatitis, mainly) have resulted in lower numbers of PTX performed in the US.

The pancreas is a vulnerable organ when compared to other abdominal solid organs. Pre-donation factors (e.g. older age, obesity, alcohol, cardiovascular disease) and intra-donation factors (e.g. retrieval damage (softer organ), warm ischemia in DCD organs) make the pancreatic graft more prone to damage during the preservation and transport phases. The pancreas donor risk index (PDRI) was developed by Axelrod et al. to be used at the time of offering to predict graft survival. The strongest risk factors were found to be donor age, BMI, DCD status, black race and cerebrovascular accident as the cause of death. Fatty infiltration is more likely in donors with BMI >35 kg/m^2 and is detrimental by causing impaired microcirculation and consequently increased risk of thrombosis and post-reperfusion pancreatitis. Donor of age >60 years and BMI >30 are unlikely to be used by most transplant centers.

Similar to other organs, brain stem death status is detrimental to the pancreas through the mechanisms of the *cathecolaminic storm*. Reduced recovery along with *in vitro* and *in vivo* function of islets from brain-dead donor rats compared with non-brain-dead is well documented. In a clinical setting, the yield of islets from DCD pancreata was 12.6% higher than from DBD donors and, expectedly, correlated negatively with warm ischemia time. However, DCD pancreata remain high risk organs mainly due to the damage sustained during the warm ischemia phase in the donor and the subsequent increased susceptibility to ischemia reperfusion injury which potentially can lead to early graft loss from graft pancreatitis and/or thrombosis.

Donor to recipient size matching is less important compared to liver transplantation. The main objective is to provide the recipient with a sufficient beta cell volume and therefore extreme mismatches are often avoided. Age also correlates negatively with graft function and survival. Many transplant centers set 50 years as the cut-off for considering donors for pancreas donation, however all donors are evaluated on a case by case basis and old donors can be used if there are no other associated risk factors. Pancreas from donors >40 years of age have a 91% increased risk of mortality when transplanted into recipients >40 years as revealed by an analysis of the Scientific Registry of Transplant Recipients. The detrimental effect of age also increases kidney graft loss in SPK. The role of HLA mismatch in PTX is not as obvious as in KTX where graft survival is clearly influenced by HLA mismatch. The largest study to date on this topic showed an increased risk of acute rejection especially in PTA rather than SPK, when HLA-B or -DR mismatches were present. This, however, did not translate into worse graft or patient survival, probably because of improved immunosuppression and management of acute rejection. In the UK organs are not allocated according to HLA match but this is factored in when considering accrual of points (vide infra). In the UK a donor pancreas is allocated to a recipient based on points (TPS, total points score) accrued in a National waiting list. These points are based on clinically relevant donor (BMI), patient (dialysis time, waiting time) and transplant related factors (total HLA mismatch, sensitization, travel time-ischemia, donor/recipient age match). A pancreas that comes from a donor where it may be used as part as a multivisceral transplant (liver/pancreas or small bowel/pancreas) is not included in the normal allocation protocol. What is also unique is that donor pancreas are also offered to patients on the National islet transplant waiting list. Generally speaking recipients need to be blood group compatible and blood group O donors, in most cases go to blood group O recipients; the exception to this rule are highly sensitized blood group A, B and AB recipients who can then receive a blood group O donor in order to minimize waiting time and risk of dying on the waiting list. Sensitization points are also accrued based on a calculated reaction frequency. We also have a pancreas fast track scheme if the pancreas is deemed unsuitable in the operating room or by a member of the transplant team/retrieval surgeon, 4 centers have already turned the pancreas down (DBD) – 3 for DCD, and finally the pancreas has not been accepted at the time of knife to skin time.

3.4   Preoperative Workup

All patients who may be candidates for pancreas transplantation in the North East of England are evaluated in the assessment clinic. Inclusion criteria and contraindications are listed in Table 3.1.

Preoperative workup (Table 3.2) includes a multidisciplinary evaluation and a final consultation with a surgeon, nephrologist and a diabetes physician. All options for PTX are discussed including the alternative option of ITX.

3.5   Surgical Technique

There has been considerable variation in the technical aspects of pancreas implantation with over 50 variations described. Some techniques were favored in the past (e.g. bladder drainage to manage exocrine secretions) and are less often adopted whilst others have been abandoned completely (e.g. gluing of the pancreatic duct).

Before implantation the pancreatic graft requires back-table preparation to remove any redundant tissue (e.g. fat,) and prepare the vascular conduit. During preparation the spleen is eventually removed but can be used as a handle to manipulate the graft, the root of the mesentery and the

TABLE 3.1 Inclusion criteria and contraindications to pancreas and islet transplantation

Inclusion criteria for pancreas transplantation:

Insulin dependent type I diabetes (or phenotypically so, defined by clinical history and undetectable serum c-peptide)

Type II diabetes (older age at onset, absence of DKA, and delayed use of insulin) may also be considered if insulin requirement <1 U/kg/24 h (ideally <0.8 U/kg). Detectable c-peptide does not preclude pancreas transplantation

Age typically less than 50

Body Mass Index (BMI) <30 kg/m^2

Satisfactory cardiovascular assessment

Progressive chronic kidney disease (CKD). Assessment should begin when eGFR is 30 ml/min, or if dialysis is anticipated within 18 months.

Simultaneous pancreas kidney (SPK) transplantation: Assessment should begin when eGFR <30 ml/min with the aim of listing patients when eGFR <15 ml/min. The presence of life threatening complications of diabetes (in addition to CKD) is not required to justify SPK. However, when such complications are present (see below) patients with any CKD may be considered for SPK transplantation.

Pancreas Transplant Alone (PTA): For patients without significant renal disease but with life threatening complications of diabetes, including:

Hypoglycemic unawareness, requiring frequent third-party intervention

Hypoglycemia leading to frequent hypoglycemic convulsions

'Brittle' diabetes, not responsive to intensive medical therapy (usually including a trial of pump therapy)

Measured GFR >60 ml/mim

Absence of proteinuria (microalbuminuria may be acceptable)

TABLE 3.1 (continued)

Pancreas After Kidney Transplant (PAK):

> May be considered for any patient meeting criteria for SPK or PTA who have already received a successful kidney transplant.

> PAK is most common after (pre-emptive) LD transplantation

> There is no requirement for a specific GFR

Inclusion criteria for islet transplantation alone

> Severe life threatening hypoglycaemia resistant to conventional therapy in C peptide negative patients [≥1 event over the preceding 12 months requiring assistance to actively administer carbohydrate, glucagon or other resuscitative actions] despite optimized conventional management

Contraindications for islet transplantation

> Insulin resistance (insulin requirement >0.7 U/kg to achieve HbA1c <9.0%),

> Body weight >80 kg

> Any contraindications to immunosuppression therapy [including impaired renal function with isotopic GFR <60 mL/min/1.73 m^2 or albumin excretion rate >300 mg/24 h (unless previous renal transplant)].

Contraindications for pancreas transplantation:

> Severe and non-correctable coronary artery disease

> Poor left ventricular function (based on functional capacity)

> Myocardial infarction within last 6 months.

> Poor prognosis cerebrovascular disease

> Ongoing substance abuse (drug or alcohol)

> Major ongoing psychiatric illness including anorexia.

> Significant history of non-compliance

(continued)

TABLE 3.1 (continued)

Active infection or malignancy excluding treated localized skin malignancy

Ongoing heavy tobacco use (cardiovascular risk)

Recurrent urinary tract infections or urological dysfunction (contraindication to bladder drained PTA/ PAK)

Severe gastroparesis (relative)

TABLE 3.2 Preoperative assessment for pancreas transplantation

Laboratory evaluation

Full blood count with differential and coagulation studies.
Thrombophilia screen (if any history of venous thrombosis).
Routine biochemistry
Mineral metabolism, including PTH
Glycosylated hemoglobin (HbA1c)
Serum lipids (triglycerides, cholesterol, HDL, LDL)
Virology (HIV, Hepatitis B & C, CMV, EBV)
ABO blood group, HLA tissue type and antibody screen

Endocrine tests

Insulin c-peptide
TFT & random cortisol
Coeliac Serology (IgA endomyseal and TTG antibody)
Islet cell and GAD 65 antibodies
T cell autoreactivity testing

Chest X-ray

Cardiology evaluation

Resting twelve-lead electrocardiogram
Resting echocardiography
    In asymptomatic patients, either myocardial perfusion scan
    with stress, or stress echocardiography
    In symptomatic patients, or those with abnormal stress
    imaging, coronary angiography
Annual review (history and 12 lead ECG, with repeated stress
testing only if clinically indicated)

TABLE 3.2 (continued)

Peripheral Vascular Assessment

Clinical examination of peripheral pulses
Duplex scanning of the pelvis and lower limbs
CT or MR angiogram if previous transplant or abnormal
duplex
Carotid duplex if symptomatic or bruit

Diabetic Evaluation

Insulin regime and diabetic control
Hypoglycemia and hypoglycemic awareness
Autonomic symptoms
Retinal Photography & report from local Ophthalmology
service (retinopathy should be quiescent or adequately
treated).
Foot and neuropathy evaluation

Gastrointestinal Tract Evaluation

History of vomiting, dysphagia, diarrhea
Upper gastrointestinal endoscopy, barium meal, transit
studies

Urinary Tract Evaluation

MSU
Post-void residual volume by USS
Urodynamics if clinical evidence bladder dysfunction
Sexual function documentation

Anesthetic Evaluation

Routine anesthetic assessment
Cardiopulmonary exercise testing

distal end of the superior mesenteric vessels are stapled off
or reinforced with a non absorbable suture. The duodenum
is shortened with the aim of keeping a well vascularized
segment which is functional to the drainage of the exocrine
secretion. Care must be taken not to cut it too short for different reasons: the risk of "pinching" the ampulla; a too short

duodenal segment leaves no options in case of reintervention for fistula, anastomotic break-down, and need to refashion the duodeno-jejunal anastomosis. The pancreas has a dual arterial system from the superior mesenteric artery (SMA) for the cephalic portion (head) and the splenic artery (SA) for the body and tail. The origins of the two arteries are implanted on a Y-shaped arterial graft obtained from the iliac arteries of the same donor so that, at the time of graft implantation, only one arterial anastomosis is required (Fig. 3.1). When the liver is not retrieved, the Y graft reconstruction is not required as the celiac axis can be used as the only arterial anastomosis, providing arterial blood supply through the common hepatic and gastroduodenal artery (GDA), and the splenic artery. A variation which avoids the use of the Y-graft has been described, anastomosing the distal end of the SMA to the splenic artery. Then the proximal SMA is used for implantation instead of the iliac Y-graft. Although various modifications have been described, the Y-graft technique remains by far the most utilized technique.

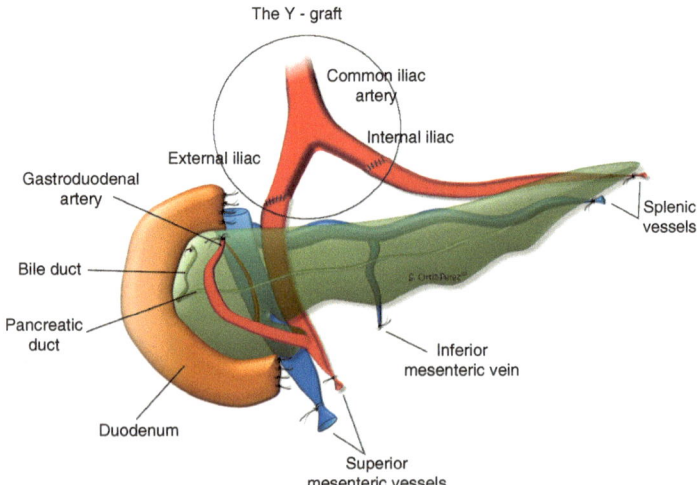

FIGURE 3.1 Pancreatic graft as prepared for implantation using arterial iliac Y-graft

The implantation starts with a midline laparotomy down to the pubis, more or less extended above the umbilicus depending on the body shape. The pancreas is implanted in the right iliac fossa but variations are common including being head up under the liver or head down towards the bladder. Exposure of the iliac axis and distal vena cava is required. The small bowel and right colon are mobilized with a Cattel-Braasch maneuver (similarly to a retrieval procedure, but without the need to extend it as much cranially). The graft can be placed more or less retroperitoneally depending on the extension of the Cattel-Braasch maneuver and the possibility to cover it with the mobilized "right mesocolon". To make the duodenal segment intraperitoneal, an incision through the mesocolon allows to reach the jejunum for the enteric drained implantation. The arterial Y-graft is anastomosed end-to side to the common iliac artery. For the venous drainage there are two possibilities: (1) systemic drainage, with the graft portal vein (PV) anastomosed end-to-side to either the common iliac vein or the distal vena cava (our preferred choice) (Fig. 3.2); (2) portal drainage, with the graft PV directly anastomosed to the recipient superior mesenteric vein (SMV) (Fig. 3.3). For portal drainage the pancreas has to be placed head up and the recipient's SMV is exposed by dissecting the root of the mesentery, after the right colon is mobilized medially, and the anastomosis is in an end-to-side fashion.

PV drainage of pancreas grafts mimics the venous flow of the native pancreas and is therefore considered more "physiologic", causing less peripheral hyperinsulinemia and also a possible immunologic advantage has been observed in experimental studies, as compared to systemic drainage. If this translates into a clinical advantage is not clear. A large case series and then a meta-analysis demonstrated equivalence between the two techniques and the systemic drainage remains more commonly utilized.

Depending on the type of exocrine drainage, the pancreas is placed head up if the graft duodenum is anastomosed to the recipient's jejunum (Figs. 3.2 and 3.3) or head down if the

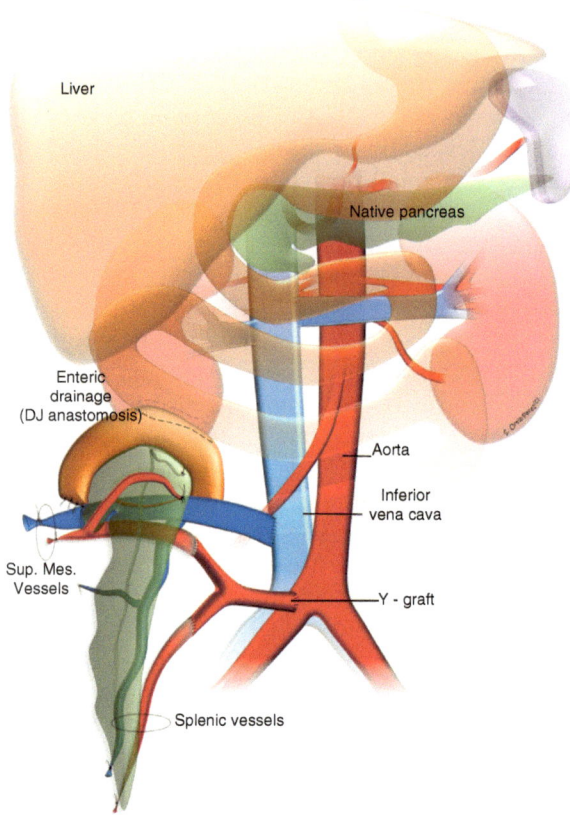

FIGURE 3.2 Pancreas transplant with enteric drainage of exocrine secretions and systemic venous drainage

duodenum is anastomosed to the bladder (Fig. 3.4). (Although head up grafts mean the venous anastomosis does not orientate laterally as it does when placed head down and some believe this may increase portal vein thrombosis rates but has not been proven in large datasets). Our personal preference for SPK in Newcastle is enteric drainage with the pancreas sitting head up with an anastomosis to the upper jejunum which

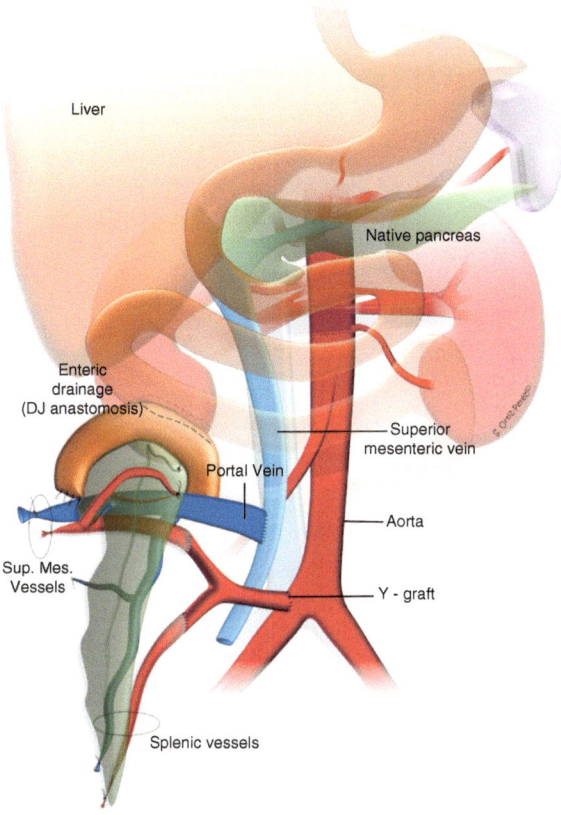

FIGURE 3.3 Pancreas transplant with enteric drainage of exocrine secretions and portal venous drainage

is thicker and more vascular than the ileum. We do not use a Roux-en-Y but create the anastomosis through a defect in the right colonic mesentery to help tether the colon back in its original position. We also remove the appendix so as to reduce a confounding factor of potential pancreatitis. We also prefer to do the bowel anastomosis in two layers with an absorbable suture on the mucosa and a non-absorbable suture on the outer wall (serosa). There is a range of opinion, we prefer prolene as it may have benefits if there is a leak although this is not evi-

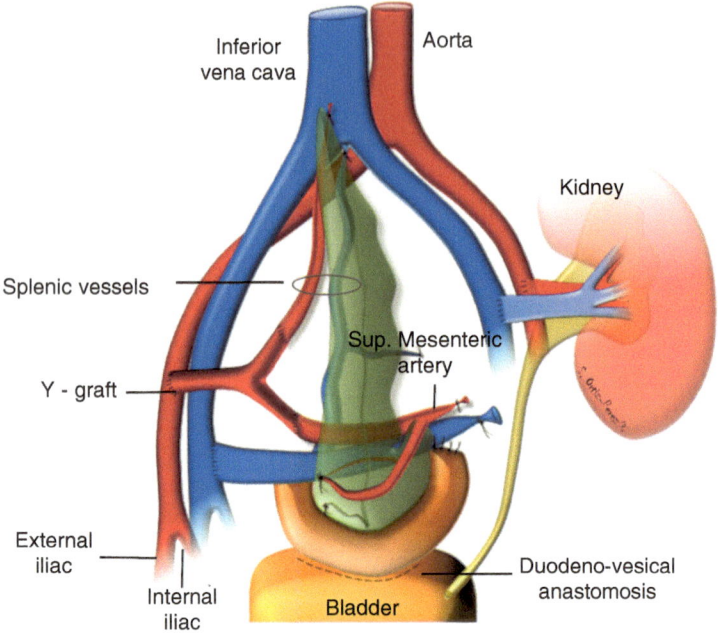

FIGURE 3.4 Simultaneous pancreas-kidney transplantation with bladder drainage of pancreatic exocrine secretion

dence based and others would argue this may increase the risk of fistulation but again there is no evidence for this. Especially in PTA and PAK, where indirect signs of rejection cannot be obtained from the kidney graft, bladder drainage allows detection of early rejection by a decline in urinary amylase concentration that precedes irreversible hyperglycemia. In addition, enteric drainage can create a contamination of the abdominal cavity with bowel content, which is of concern especially in the context of heavy immunosuppression such as that adopted in the past but these theoretical risks have not been proven. Duodenal leak is easier to manage with bladder drainage by prolonged catheterization, while some surgeons establish the enteric drainage through a Roux-en-Y isolated limb to avoid fasting patients with leaks however a Roux en Y is not critical and many surgeons do not use them. Because there is relatively high concordance in histologic signs of rejection in the duodenum and the pancreatic parenchyma, another advantage with bladder drainage is a relatively easy access to the graft duodenum which can be biopsied via cystoscopy. Boggi et al. proposed to anastomose the graft to the recipient's duodenum to establish a similar ease of access to the graft endoscopically, however in case a transplantectomy is required, the recipient is left with a breach in the native duodenum which is complex to manage. As demonstrated more recently, enteroscopy can be used to reach the duodenal graft mucosa and some centers have adopted it as their routine practice.

Altogether, with the evolution of immunosuppression and widespread application of PTX, enteric drainage has been favored because of the more physiologic dismissal of the pancreatic enzymes and bicarbonates inside the bowel instead of the bladder where they can cause chemical cystitis, urethral stenosis, dehydration and metabolic acidosis. Conversion from bladder to enteric drainage has been described in up to 45% of recipients and some centers adopt bladder drainage in isolated PTX and switch to enteric drainage after the first year post-transplantation, when the risk of rejection starts to decrease, unless they are tolerating well the bladder drained pancreas.

Most of the pancreas transplants are performed together with a kidney transplant. The kidney graft is placed in the left iliac fossa. Despite the midline laparotomy approach, there is still a possibility to place it extraperitoneally by dissecting the peritoneum to the left of the *linea alba* down to the iliac fossa, creating a sort of "extraperitoneal pocket". Such technical solution shares the same advantages of solitary kidney transplantation which is normally extraperitoneal (e.g. ease of access for percutaneous biopsy, maintaining graft complications confined, not involving intraperitoneal organs, etc.).

3.6 Post-Operative Management

For our patients we assess fluid replacement frequently as well as the need for dialysis if there is evidence of delayed graft function of the kidney. Nasogastric drainage usually continues to day 5 in enteric drained PTX. We also start nasojejunal feeding slowly at 10–75 ml/h (max rate). Routine management includes a chest X-ray to check central line placement, daily input/output charts, blood pressure monitoring, temperature, pulse oximetry, and monitor urine output for delayed graft function of kidney.

We aim to maintain systolic blood pressure to around 120 mmHg and give colloids/albumin/0.9% saline solution as appropriate. We take daily full blood count, kidney and liver function tests, electrolytes,, clotting, serum amylase and lipase, drain amylase and lipase, blood glucose and thromboelastogram (TEG).

Anti-hypertensives (e.g. beta blockers) medications due to ischemic heart disease should be continuedas well as subcutaneous Tinzaparin 3500 units and TED stockings (if no diabetic ulcers). Therapeutic dose of heparin may need to be added dependent on TEG status as well as day 5 MRI scan. Sodium docusate via nasogastric tube avoids hardening of stool (100 mg three times daily) as well as gastric mucosa protection with a proton pump inhibitor. For bladder drained PTX, sodium bicarbonate 1300 mg BD is needed to prevent metabolic acidosis. We may also use subcutaneous Octreotide 200 mcg three times daily to reduce pancreatic secretions (optional) if we suspect a pancreatic leak. Fluconazole 200 mg PO for 7 days prophylaxis continues if cultures become positive or iliac vessel culture media is positive. Antimicrobial prophylaxis includes trimethoprim/sulfamethoxazole 80/400 mg orally, piperacillin/tazobactam 4.5 g three times daily i.v. for 5 days, simvastatin 20 mg or their regular statin, trough tacrolimus levels, aspirin 75 mg if not already prescribed. Doppler ultrasound of the kidney and pancreas to evaluate perfusion although in the latter a day 5 MRI of the pancreas and vessels is always done. Pancreas transplants often start working immediately, however there can sometimes be a surge of inappropriate insulin secretion needing large volumes of intravenous dextrose. Continue insulin/dextrose infusion as above (10 units actrapid insulin in 500 ml 10% dextrose infused at 80 ml/h). Prolonged hyperglycemia can be damaging to a pancreas graft.

3.6.1   CMV Prophylaxis

With the increasing use of antibody therapy and profound immunodepletion this is very important. Transplant coordinators will carefully document donor and recipient status. Transplantation of a positive CMV donor organ IgG + (D+) into a CMV negative recipient IgG - (R-) will require Valganciclovir. If the patient has antibody therapy (e.g. Alemtuzumab), then D+ into R+ should also have Valganciclovir. Valganciclovir dose has to be adjusted according to renal function.

3.6.2   Management Main Complications

3.6.2.1   Pancreatic Leak

Management of a pancreatic leak depends on whether the pancreas is bladder drained or enterically drained, with leaks being more common in the latter. The incidence is between 5–18%. In most cases they can be managed conservatively. Octreotide is sometimes used as prophylaxis depending on the preference of the surgeon. They most commonly present during post-operative days 5–12. Generally, bladder drained leaks are less serious. To minimize leaks some units advocate two layered anastomotic techniques or the use of non-absorbable sutures as previously described. Leaks may also be caused by ulceration from CMV and ischemia. Mild bladder drained leaks can usually be treated by prolonged bladder catheterization. Early leaks are usually from the duodenoenteric or duodenovesical anastomosis, late leaks are usually from the staple lines of the duodenal stump. Signs and symptoms include abdominal pain/distension/vomiting or high NG aspirates with a temperature and even peritonitis in severe cases. Investigations would include raised creatinine (if primary renal function), high amylase/lipase in the abdominal drains (>1000), raised serum amylase (in 50%), reduced urinary amylase, a raised WCC, blood cultures, urine culture and a CMV screen. An abdominal CT scan is essential to identify any fluid collection for percutaneous drainage and also for microbiology.

If the patient has peritonitis the management is surgical. Most enteric drained leaks can be managed by appropriate antibiotics and percutaneous drainage of any abdominal collection. Bowel rest with parenteral nutrition and intravenous octreotide can also help. Infected, persistent leaks may require re-laparotomy. Prophylaxis with subcutaneous Octreotide 200 mcg TDS to be stopped at day 5, or therapeutic Octreotide 500 mcg in 50 mL 0.9% saline (start infusion at 5 ml/h increasing to 10 ml/h if no benefit) can be used. Long-term octreotide formulations are available; Lanreotide (Somatuline) Autogel 60 mg every 3 weeks by deep subcutaneous injection. Side effects include gastrointestinal disturbance such as bloating, nausea, vomiting, diarrhea, steatorrhea and abdominal cramps, hyperglycaemia and abnormal LFT's.

3.6.2.2   Graft Pancreatitis

Pancreas transplantation is perceived as a high risk procedure because of the patients being diabetic but mortality rates are low. The graft (more so the acinar tissue) is prone to ischemia reperfusion injury which can lead to pancreatitis and thrombosis. Graft pancreatitis is also common while enteric anastomotic leaks and intra-abdominal sepsis occur less often. Graft pancreatitis is more common in DCD pancreas transplants because the acinar tissue is more susceptible to ischemia. Allograft pancreatitis can be of varying degrees of severity and altogether affects 40% of patients but only in some cases is clinically relevant and needs an intervention (e.g. drainage). When severe, graft pancreatitis can be a life-threatening condition and can cause graft dysfunction, prolonged hospital stay and further complications, in the worse scenario graft pancreatectomy. It usually presents with abdominal pain, tenderness over the graft, fever, vomiting or diarrhea. In most cases no obvious cause can be found; it can be attributable to urinary reflux, urinary infections or bladder outlet obstruction in bladder drained grafts. Therefore, bladder catherization can be useful. Patients may need percutaneous drainage of abdominal collections or re-laparotomy and washout if not accessible radiologically. Treatment often entails bowel rest, intravenous fluids, antibiotics if septic and percutaneous drainage.

3.6.2.3   Pseudoaneursyms

Visceral transplant pseudoaneurysm formation is a rare but potentially life threatening complication with a multifactorial etiology including; surgical technique, infection, postoperative anastomotic/bile leak and pancreatitis. Fungal infection is the most common organism. Prophylactic antibiotics or antifungals should be used if a positive culture is found in the transport fluid of the iliac vessels or the pancreas itself. Clinical presentation is also highly variable ranging from asymptomatic (detected on routine imagine follow up) to life threatening (acute rupture). Pancreatic transplant pseudoaneurysms are rare. The treatment of pseudoaneurysms remains controversial and due to its infrequent occurrence there is a paucity of published literature to support a definitive management approach. Traditional teaching has suggested that resection/reanastomosis or reconstruction with grafts can be an option. However, this is not advised in the context of acute rupture or potential presence of infection. Transplant artery ligation is another management approach that has been suggested.

Endovascular management can be considered as an alternative to surgery. The location of transplant pseudoaneurysms is critical when considering an endovascular approach. For pseudoaneurysms of the transplant artery itself away from the anastomosis, stent grafting has been shown to be a successful technique. However, when a transplant artery pseudoaneurysm involves the anastomosis or ostium, standard stent grafting is of limited value because it would involve sacrificing/covering the transplant vessel origin thereby risking the graft. In order to preserve flow into a transplant artery whilst excluding the pseudoaneurysm from blood flow, this requires stent grafting in a T configuration using a fenestration to preserve the graft vessel. There is no commercially available endovascular device designed for this purpose. Endovascular options therefore are limited to custom graft ordering or physician modification of existing equipment. As custom endovascular device manufacturing can take months, this is not a suitable option to manage the emergent nature of transplant pseudoaneurysms. Prolonged sepsis remains a problem and long-term antibiotics may be needed.

3.6.3   Immunosuppression

Pancreas transplantation requires immunosuppression not only for prevention of allograft rejection but also due to the risk of autoimmune recurrence of type 1, as observed in transplantation between identical twins.

Antibody induction therapy and maintenance with calcineurin inhibitors (CNI) and antimetabolite drugs are the mainstay of immunosuppression in PTX. Steroid avoidance or early withdrawal are commonly adopted with the aim of minimizing insulin resistance. In general, a non-diabetogenic, non-nephrotoxic and non-gastrointestinal toxic maintenance immunosuppressive regimen is desirable for all solid organ transplant recipients, but is particularly relevant in PTX. Current 1-year rates of immunological pancreas graft loss are 6.0% in PTA, 3.7% in PAK and 1.8% in SPK transplants. In general, it is now unusual to lose a graft because of immune-mediated rejection.

Pancreas grafts are more often transplanted in combination with the kidney, which makes PTX a unique challenge in the management of immunosuppression. Isolated PTX accounted for only 8% of all PTX in the UK in 2016/2017.

When performed in combination with a kidney transplant, the incidence of rejection is lower, especially in SPKs where the organs are both from the same donor, while in PTA's a more aggressive immunosuppressive approach is required and a quadruple therapy including induction antibodies and maintenance with corticosteroids (although discontinued early) are utilized by some centers. In Newcastle we adopt a steroid-free regimen (only Methylprednisolone 500 mg is given intraoperatively) with induction using Alemtuzumab (subcutaneous injection) after hemostasis has been achieved and then again on day 3. Maintenance is based on Tacrolimus 0.05 mg/kg (targeting trough levels 8–12 μg/L) and Mycophenolate Mofetil (MMF) 500 mg twice a day.

The vast majority (85–90%) of pancreas transplant recipients receive antibody induction which can be based on lymphocyte depleting or non-depleting IL-2 receptor blockers antibodies. More than 70% receive depleting T-cell antibody induction, usually with rabbit anti-thymocyte globulin (rATG). This approach allows steroid avoidance or early withdrawal and reduces the incidence of acute rejection within the first 6 months. Steroid free recipients treated with alemtuzumab reported lower rates of cytomegalovirus (CMV) infections as compared to those receiving rATG. Although antibody induction may result in lower rates of acute rejection, no specific induction strategy has been associated with improved intermediate-term outcomes in PTX.

The most common maintenance regime is Tacrolimus combined with Mycophenolate acid derivates; the use of Cyclosporine A (CyA) and Azathioprine (AZA) are reserved to those who develop intolerance to Tacrolimus and mycophenolate respectively. The SPK 001 trial, compared Tacrolimus against CyA, revealing similar patient and kidney allograft survival at 1 year, with pancreas survival being significantly higher with tacrolimus (91 versus 75%). At 3 years, patient and kidney survival rates remained similar, whilst pancreas survival remained significantly higher with tacrolimus (90 versus 72%). Pancreas allograft loss due to thrombosis was increased with CyA (10 versus 2 patients).

Lower rates and longer time to first kidney allograft rejection in SPK have been reported in a prospective randomized trial with MMF against AZA. In patients with gastrointestinal symptoms (often reported in type 1 diabetics with gastroparesis) may benefit from mycophenolate sodium before considering switching to AZA.

The use of mammalian target of Rapamycin (mTOR) immunosuppressants against MMF in combination with Tacrolimus was the object of the Euro-SPK-002 study At 1 year, there were more study withdrawal in the Rapamycin group compared to the MMF group, due to toxicity, although more than 60% of those patients were rejection free at 1 year. Serum creatinine level was significantly lower in the Rapamycin group from month 2, however there were higher incidence of hyperlipidemia, delayed wound healing, lymphocele or hernia. The results of a 10 year-long randomized single center trial showed Rapamycin (Sirolimus) in combination with Tacrolimus was better tolerated (i.e. less gastrointestinal side effects and need to withhold medications) and more effective than the combination Tacrolimus/MMF (probably due to MMF being withheld more often because of gastrointestinal side effects). Overall, the patient and allograft survival were equivalent.

For the treatment of acute cell-mediated rejection without a substantial vascular component (Banff <2A on renal biopsy) or empirically, in our Center we utilize methylprednisolone 500 mg for three consecutive days. For steroid-resistant cell-mediated rejection, or for significant cell-mediated vascular rejection (Banff 2B or worse), we use rATG.

3.6.4   Thrombosis and Anticoagulation

Bleeding and thrombosis are the most frequent early-onset surgical complications with a reported incidence of % and 3 to 17% respectively. Vascular thrombosis is the main cause of early non-immunological, graft loss. Pancreatic grafts harbor an intrinsic tendency towards thrombosis due to the high capacitance, low-flow state that ensues through the splenic and superior mesenteric veins after disconnection of the spleen and the small bowel from the graft. In addition, type 1 diabetics suffer an inherent hypercoagulable status. However, immediately after surgery, routine systemic anticoagulation is controversial because of an increased bleeding risk. Venous thrombosis often leads to catastrophic consequences unless it is identified. Early classic signs are abdominal pain, hyperglycemia, rising lactate, a fall in hemoglobin. Unfortunately, this often needs graft pancreatectomy but in rare circumstances it can be salvaged by endovascular thrombectomy if there is sufficient run off in the vessels. Hemorrhage after PTX is the leading cause for relaparotomy which is a risk factor for graft loss.

In our Center, we use Dextran 40 and low molecular weight heparin (LMWH) during the first 24–48 h postoperatively. Thromboelastography (TEG) is used to identify hypercoagulable status and if so, intravenous heparin is started, similarly described by other centers. All patients have a CT angiogram at day 5 to exclude any developing thrombus. The infusion rate is regulated using anti factor Xa monitoring. Aspirin and/or LMWH are used for maintenance while oral anticoagulants are reserved for high thrombotic risk recipients.

3.7   Outcomes

3.7.1   Patient and Graft Survival

More than 50,000 PTX have been reported to the International Pancreatic Transplant Registry (IPTR) (> 29,000 from the United States and >19,000 from other countries), and patient survival rates have improved significantly over time in all categories of recipients. The most recent data analysis from the US population within the IPTR showed the following figures:

– One-year patient survival rates have been over 95% in 2005–09 and over 96% in 2010–14. Five-year patient survival is close to 90% for all categories of recipients. Cardiac or cerebro-vascular (CCV) diseases and infections are the leading causes of early and late recipient death, which are seen most frequently in the first 3 months posttransplant, but also remain the principal causes of death later on.

– Graft survival rates are of 89%, 84% and 83% at 1 year respectively for SPK, PAK and PTA transplanted in the era 2010 to 2014, which constitutes a significant improvement for SPK and PAK pancreatic grafts when compared to the previous era 2005 to 2009.

– The main cause of graft loss during the first 3 months posttransplant for primary transplants is early technical problems in all 3 categories followed by death with a functioning graft (DWFG). Technical losses are higher in PTA than in SPK. Between 3 months and 1 year after transplant, DWFG becomes the most frequent reason for graft failure in SPK while acute immunological problems peak for PTA. Infections account for 12% of graft losses in all 3 categories. Chronic rejection is the most relevant cause of graft loss in PTA and to a lesser extent in PAK while DWFG is prevalent in SPK.
– Older donors, CCV as cause of death and extended preservation times are associated with significantly higher rates of graft loss. This effect is more marked in the pancreas graft than on the kidney graft.

Data from the National Health System Blood and Transplant in the United Kingdom show a risk adjusted patient and pancreatic graft survival respectively of 97% and 88% at 1 year and 89% and 78% at 5 years after deceased donor pancreas transplantation of any type.

The definition of graft failure remains a matter of debate: some centers consider it as lack of C-peptide whilst others accept insulin dependence. The consensus report from the IPITA/EPITA opinion leaders workshop highlighted the use of insulin or other anti-hyperglycemic therapy following pancreas or islet transplantation is not synonymous with graft loss or failure, as patients may require low doses of exogenous insulin- or other glucose-lowering agents to maintain glycemic control in the non-diabetic range, which is only possible to achieve when a portion of the insulin requirement is provided endogenously from a functioning graft. They categorized beta cell graft function (either solid organ or islets) based on HbA1c levels, number of episodes of severe hypoglycemia, insulin requirements and C-peptide levels. Success of a transplant was considered not only if the recipient is completely insulin free but also when insulin requirements post transplantation are <50% of pre-transplant levels.

3.7.2 Effects on Diabetes-Related Complications

After a phase of skepticism regarding reversal of some of the secondary diabetic complications after pancreas transplantation, diabetes related complications have been shown to stabilize or improve after SPK. Improvements have been observed in diabetic nephropathy, neuropathy, gastroparesis, retinopathy, cardiac function and sexual function in some form or another. In patients with diabetic nephropathy, reversal of glomerular and cortical lesions from diabetic nephropathy has been reported. One study showed almost complete normalization of glomerular lesions in native kidneys 10 years post-transplant.

Less data on the evolution of secondary complications are available for recipients of PTA. A reduction in cardiovascular risk factors and improved cardiac function has been demonstrated in patients with T1DM.

Although PAK has lower pancreas graft survival than SPK, PAK improves kidney graft survival in the long term and the benefit is more pronounced if the gap between the two transplants is less than 1 year.

Beneficial effects have been reported on all types of diabetic neuropathy (sensory, motor, and autonomic), using different methodologies, including clinical scores of symptoms, physical examination and sensory testing, nerve conduction studies and autonomic function tests.

3.7.3 Survival Benefit

The survival benefit of SPK against KTX alone in diabetic patients has been demonstrated in several studies. A large analysis of 13,467 patients from the US Scientific Renal Transplant Registry and the US Renal Data System, showed the greatest longevity (23.4 years) for SPK recipients followed by those who received only a living donor kidney transplant (20.9 years) and recipients of a kidney transplant from a deceased donor (12.8 years).

In recipients of PTA with brittle diabetes, the mortality rate at 4 years is lower than that of candidates on the waiting list (9.5% versus 12.7% respectively). This gap between wait listed patients and transplant recipients is far bigger in SPK recipients.

Improved long-term results with PTX has changed the perception of such intervention from one which only improves quality of life to one which extends life too.

3.8   Future Perspectives

A reduction in the number of PTX seems to be a global trend in the last decade. The genesis of this phenomenon is multifactorial and includes improved glycemic control using continuous insulin pumps, the relative stagnation of PTX from the technical point of view in the last 30 years, the perceived high risk of morbidity and non-insignificant perioperative mortality associated with PTX itself. Having to use more marginal high risk donors (older, more obese, DCD) and type 2 diabetes has also been a contributing factor along with competition with islet transplant alone. Such a trend confines PTX to a highly selected group of patients, using more stringent selection criteria for donors, minimizing the risk of early graft failures but at the price of excluding a wider cohort of diabetic patients with advanced disease.

The ongoing technological evolution allows one to expect more refined systems of continuous glucose monitoring and exogenous insulin infusion through closed loop systems.

Stem cell based treatments have a great potential once issues such as large scale production of functional beta cells and techniques to implant them with long-term function will continue to be addressed. Stem cell research has allowed the transformation of embryonic stem cells into pancreatic β-cells. The in vitro generation of functional β-cells from human induced pluripotent stem cells derived from patients with T1DM can correct hyperglycemia in mice. However, stem cells may possibly continue to proliferate in an uncontrolled manner after implantation in patients.

Gene therapy has the potential of eliminating diabetes either by eliminating processes which cause insulin depletion or by adding new pathways of insulin production. Although encouraging, it is far from appearing into clinical practice.

There is great interest in the development of synthetic and biological scaffolds from decellularized animals or discarded human organs which can be used as an extracellular matrix in the hope to rebuild whole organs. Such an experimental field is still in an embryonic phase however it is extremely promising.

Xenotransplantation with porcine islets is a promising approach to overcome the shortage of human donors. A clinical trial of intra-peritoneal encapsulated porcine islets in non-immunosuppressed diabetic patients was undertaken in New Zealand. The study consisted of the transplantation of pig islets by laparoscopy into the peritoneal cavity in 14 patients with unstable T1DM, without any immunosuppressive therapy. There was an improvement in the number of episodes of hypoglycemia unawareness, although not statistically significant (probably also due to the small number of cases). Porcine non-capsulated ITX in primates (and humans) induce an immediate inflammatory response which causes early graft rejection despite immunosuppression, while encapsulated islets do not require immunosuppression but are less reactive to glycemic fluctuations.

3.9   Additional Professional Skills for the Surgeon

Pancreas transplantation is a composite procedure, the success of which depends on innumerable factors including fine surgical skills and careful planning. The greatest attention must be paid to avoid even the smallest damage to the graft, starting from the retrieval, all the way through the back-table preparation, ending after the implantation. Manipulation of the pancreas causes acinar cells disruption, increasing the risk of post-operative graft pancreatitis and thrombosis. Pancreatic capsule tears can cause prolonged – potentially untreatable - exocrine secretion leaks.

Pancreas retrieval is commonly regarded as the last skill to acquire for the retrieval surgeon in training. Some centers send their pancreatic surgeons to retrieve the graft, which allows more warm-phase dissection, better control of the hemostasis of the graft (thanks to the possibility of identifying and controlling potential sources of bleeding while still on the heartbeat) and quicker back-table preparation. In countries such as the United Kingdom where a centralized retrieval system is in place, retrieval surgeons are more often not dedicated pancreatic surgeons and therefore they carry out most of the dissection of the pancreas during the cold phase in order to minimize the risk of unintended injuries. Retrieval surgeons are asked to "dissect away" from the organ capsule, as capsular injuries might make the organ unusable because of potential leakage of pancreatic fluid which is extremely difficult to treat. Even when retrieving the pancreas for islet transplantation, care must be taken to keep the organ intact, as capsular tears can jeopardize the process of islets extraction.

Peculiar vascular anatomy requires mastering various anastomosis techniques for the arterial reconstruction. Pancreas back-table surgery is typically the lengthiest of all abdominal organs. The surgeon must be confident and efficient enough to keep a quick pace and reduce excessive cold ischemia time. Implantation more often consists of pancreas and kidney transplantation and the surgeon has to acquire skills not only in managing potentially complex vascular scenarios but also in bladder and bowel reconstruction techniques. In addition, retransplantation of either pancreas or kidney are not uncommon situations in patients with complex history of T1DM who want to ameliorate their expectancy and quality of life. Pancreas transplant surgeons are required to be confident in explanting failed grafts, handling previously dissected blood vessels and in some cases "making space" for more organs to be transplanted (e.g. recipients with more 3 or 4 heterotopic organs in their abdomen because of SPK retransplantation and no explant of the previously failed grafts).

3.10   Conclusion

Pancreas transplantation has evolved greatly since it was first performed in 1966, to the point of becoming the gold standard treatment for type 1 diabetic patients with uremia. It is the most durable solution to maintain long-term euglycemia and halt and to some extent reverse diabetes related systemic complications. It has been extended to selected type 2 diabetic patients and it has the ability to resolve hypoglycemic unawareness in brittle diabetes.

Despite all of this, little evolution and a change in the donor habitus combined with high morbidity rates have resulted in it pancreas transplantation being an endangered procedure with real fear of extinction.

Until islet transplantation becomes more resource efficient and durable combined with continued technological advances, pancreas transplantation will remain the best option for diabetic patients with severe complications and poor glycemic control.

Bibliography

1. Asher JF, Wilson CH, Talbot D, Manas DM, Williams R, White SA. Successful endovascular salvage of a pancreatic graft after a venous thrombosis: case report and literature review. Exp Clin Transplant. 2013;11(4):375–8.
2. Axelrod D, Leventhal JR, Gallon LG, Parker MA, Kaufman DB. Reduction of CMV disease with steroid-free immunosuppresssion in simultaneous pancreas-kidney transplant recipients. Am J Transplant. 2005;5(6):1423–9.
3. Axelrod DA, Sung RS, Meyer KH, Wolfe RA, Kaufman DB. Systematic evaluation of pancreas allograft quality, outcomes and geographic variation in utilization. Am J Transplant. 2010;10(4):837–45.
4. Becker BN, Brazy PC, Becker YT, Odorico JS, Pintar TJ, Collins BH, et al. Simultaneous pancreas-kidney transplantation reduces excess mortality in type 1 diabetic patients with end-stage renal disease. Kidney Int. 2000;57(5):2129–35.

5. Bergenstal RM, Tamborlane WV, Ahmann A, Buse JB, Dailey G, Davis SN, et al. Effectiveness of sensor-augmented insulin-pump therapy in type 1 diabetes. N Engl J Med. 2010;363(4):311–20.
6. Berney T, Boffa C, Augustine T, Badet L, de Koning E, Pratschke J, et al. Utilization of organs from donors after circulatory death for vascularized pancreas and islet of Langerhans transplantation: recommendations from an expert group. Transpl Int. 2016;29(7):798–806.
7. Boggi U, Amorese G, Marchetti P, Mosca F. Segmental live donor pancreas transplantation: review and critique of rationale, outcomes, and current recommendations. Clin Transpl. 2011;25(1):4–12.
8. Boggi U, Rosati CM, Marchetti P. Follow-up of secondary diabetic complications after pancreas transplantation. Curr Opin Organ Transplant. 2013;18(1):102–10.
9. Boggi U, Vistoli F, Signori S, Del Chiaro M, Campatelli A, Amorese G, et al. A technique for retroperitoneal pancreas transplantation with portal-enteric drainage. Transplantation. 2005;79(9):1137–42.
10. Brooks AM, Walker N, Aldibbiat A, Hughes S, Jones G, de Havilland J, et al. Attainment of metabolic goals in the integrated UK islet transplant program with locally isolated and transported preparations. Am J Transplant. 2013;13(12):3236–43.
11. Browne S, Gill J, Dong J, Rose C, Johnston O, Zhang P, et al. The impact of pancreas transplantation on kidney allograft survival. Am J Transplant. 2011;11(9):1951–8.
12. Burke GW, Ciancio G, Figueiro J, Buigas R, Olson L, Roth D, et al. Hypercoagulable state associated with kidney-pancreas transplantation. Thromboelastogram-directed anti-coagulation and implications for future therapy. Clin Transpl. 2004;18(4):423–8.
13. Choi JY, Jung JH, Kwon H, Shin S, Kim YH, Han DJ. Pancreas transplantation from living donors: a single center experience of 20 cases. Am J Transplant. 2016;16(8):2413–20.
14. Contreras JL, Eckstein C, Smyth CA, Sellers MT, Vilatoba M, Bilbao G, et al. Brain death significantly reduces isolated pancreatic islet yields and functionality in vitro and in vivo after transplantation in rats. Diabetes. 2003;52(12):2935–42.
15. Dholakia S, Royston E, Quiroga I, Sinha S, Reddy S, Gilbert J, et al. The rise and potential fall of pancreas transplantation. Br Med Bull. 2017;124(1):171–9.

16. Fernández-Cruz L, Astudillo E, Sanfey H, Llovera JM, Saenz A, Lopez-Boado MA, et al. Combined whole pancreas and liver retrieval: comparison between Y-iliac graft and splenomesenteric anastomosis. Transpl Int. 1992;5(1):54–6.

17. Fioretto P, Mauer M. Reversal of diabetic nephropathy: lessons from pancreas transplantation. J Nephrol. 2012;25(1):13–8.

18. Fiorina P, Vezzulli P, Bassi R, Gremizzi C, Falautano M, D'Addio F, et al. Near normalization of metabolic and functional features of the central nervous system in type 1 diabetic patients with end-stage renal disease after kidney-pancreas transplantation. Diabetes Care. 2012;35(2):367–74.

19. Goh S-K, Bertera S, Olsen P, Candiello J, Halfter W, Uechi G, et al. Perfusion-decellularized pancreas as a natural 3D scaffold for pancreatic tissue and whole organ engineering. Biomaterials. 2013;34(28):6760–72.

20. Gruessner AC, Gruessner RWG. Pancreas transplantation of US and non-US cases from 2005 to 2014 as reported to the united network for organ sharing (UNOS) and the international pancreas transplant registry (IPTR). Rev Diabet Stud RDS. 2016;13(1):35–58.

21. Gruessner AC, Laftavi MR, Pankewycz O, Gruessner RWG. Simultaneous pancreas and kidney transplantation-is it a treatment option for patients with type 2 diabetes mellitus? An analysis of the international pancreas transplant registry. Curr Diab Rep. 2017;17(6):44.

22. Kandaswamy R, Stock PG, Gustafson SK, Skeans MA, Curry MA, Prentice MA, et al. OPTN/SRTR 2016 Annual Data Report: Pancreas. Am J Transplant. 18(S1):114–71.

23. Kaufman DB, Burke GW, Bruce DS, Johnson CP, Gaber AO, Sutherland DER, et al. Prospective, randomized, multi-center trial of antibody induction therapy in simultaneous pancreas-kidney transplantation. Am J Transplant. 2003;3(7):855–64.

24. Kayler LK, Wen X, Zachariah M, Casey M, Schold J, Magliocca J. Outcomes and survival analysis of old-to-old simultaneous pancreas and kidney transplantation. Transpl Int. 2013;26(10):963–72.

25. Kelly WD, Lillehei RC, Merkel FK, Idezuki Y, Goetz FC. Allotransplantation of the pancreas and duodenum along with the kidney in diabetic nephropathy. Surgery. 1967;61(6):827–37.

26. Khaja MS, Matsumoto AH, Saad WE. Vascular complications of transplantation: part 2: pancreatic transplants. Cardiovasc Intervent Radiol. 2014;37(6):1415–9.

27. Kirchner VA, Finger EB, Bellin MD, Dunn TB, Gruessner RWG, Hering BJ, et al. Long-term outcomes for living pancreas donors in the modern era. Transplantation. 2016;100(6):1322–8.
28. Lehmann R, Graziano J, Brockmann J, Pfammatter T, Kron P, de Rougemont O, et al. Glycemic control in simultaneous islet-kidney versus pancreas-kidney transplantation in type 1 diabetes: a prospective 13-year follow-up. Diabetes Care. 2015;38(5):752–9.
29. Lin Y, Sun Z. Antiaging gene klotho attenuates pancreatic β-cell apoptosis in type 1 diabetes. Diabetes. 2015;64(12):4298–311.
30. Lombardo C, Baronti W, Amorese G, Vistoli F, Marchetti P, Boggi U. Transplantation of the pancreas. In: De Groot LJ, Chrousos G, Dungan K, Feingold KR, Grossman A, Hershman JM, et al., editors. Endotext [Internet]. South Dartmouth (MA): MDText.com, Inc.; 2000.. Available from: http://www.ncbi.nlm.nih.gov/books/NBK278979/.
31. Luan FL, Kommareddi M, Cibrik DM, Samaniego M, Ojo AO. The time interval between kidney and pancreas transplantation and the clinical outcomes of pancreas after kidney transplantation. Clin Transpl. 2012;26(3):403–10.
32. Marang-van de Mheen PJ, Nijhof HW, Khairoun M, Haasnoot A, van der Boog PJM, Baranski AG. Pancreas-kidney transplantations with primary bladder drainage followed by enteric conversion: graft survival and outcomes. Transplantation. 2008;85(4):517–23.
33. Margreiter C, Aigner F, Resch T, Berenji A-K, Oberhuber R, Sucher R, et al. Enteroscopic biopsies in the management of pancreas transplants: a proof of concept study for a novel monitoring tool. Transplantation. 2012;93(2):207–13.
34. Matsumoto S, Tan P, Baker J, Durbin K, Tomiya M, Azuma K, et al. Clinical porcine islet xenotransplantation under comprehensive regulation. Transplant Proc. 2014;46(6):1992–5.
35. Muthusamy ASR, Mumford L, Hudson A, Fuggle SV, Friend PJ. Pancreas transplantation from donors after circulatory death from the United Kingdom. Am J Transplant. 2012;12(8):2150–6.
36. Niederhaus SV, Kaufman DB, Odorico JS. Induction therapy in pancreas transplantation. Transpl Int. 2013;26(7):704–14.
37. Ojo AO, Meier-Kriesche HU, Hanson JA, Leichtman A, Magee JC, Cibrik D, et al. The impact of simultaneous pancreas-kidney transplantation on long-term patient survival. Transplantation. 2001;71(1):82–90.

38. Oliver JB, Beidas A-K, Bongu A, Brown L, Shapiro ME. A comparison of long-term outcomes of portal versus systemic venous drainage in pancreatic transplantation: a systematic review and meta-analysis. Clin Transpl. 2015;29(10):882–92.

39. Pagliuca FW, Millman JR, Gürtler M, Segel M, Van Dervort A, Ryu JH, et al. Generation of functional human pancreatic β cells in vitro. Cell. 2014;159(2):428–39.

40. Pruijm MT, de Fijter HJW, Doxiadis II, Vandenbroucke JP. Preemptive versus non-preemptive simultaneous pancreas-kidney transplantation: a single-center, long-term, follow-up study. Transplantation. 2006;81(8):1119–24.

41. Rickels MR, Schutta MH, Mueller R, Markmann JF, Barker CF, Naji A, et al. Islet cell hormonal responses to hypoglycemia after human islet transplantation for type 1 diabetes. Diabetes. 2005;54(11):3205–11.

42. Rickels MR, Stock PG, de Koning EJP, Piemonti L, Pratschke J, Alejandro R, et al. Defining outcomes for β-cell replacement therapy in the treatment of diabetes: a consensus report on the Igls criteria from the IPITA/EPITA opinion leaders workshop. Transpl Int. 2018;31(4):343–52.

43. Rudolph EN, Dunn TB, Mauer D, Noreen H, Sutherland DER, Kandaswamy R, et al. HLA-A, -B, -C, −DR, and -DQ matching in pancreas transplantation: effect on graft rejection and survival. Am J Transplant. 2016;16(8):2401–12.

44. Saudek F, Malaise J, Boucek P, Adamec M. Euro-SPK Study Group. Efficacy and safety of tacrolimus compared with cyclosporin microemulsion in primary SPK transplantation: 3-year results of the Euro-SPK 001 trial. Nephrol Dial Transplant. 2005;20(Suppl 2):ii3–10. ii62.

45. Scalea JR, Butler CC, Munivenkatappa RB, Nogueira JM, Campos L, Haririan A, et al. Pancreas transplant alone as an independent risk factor for the development of renal failure: a retrospective study. Transplantation. 2008;86(12):1789–94.

46. Scheffert JL, Taber DJ, Pilch NA, Chavin KD, Baliga PK, Bratton CF. Clinical outcomes associated with the early postoperative use of heparin in pancreas transplantation. Transplantation. 2014;97(6):681–5.

47. Shapiro AM, Lakey JR, Ryan EA, Korbutt GS, Toth E, Warnock GL, et al. Islet transplantation in seven patients with type 1 diabetes mellitus using a glucocorticoid-free immunosuppressive regimen. N Engl J Med. 2000;343(4):230–8.

48. Siskind EJ, Amodu LI, Pinto S, Akerman M, Jonsson J, Molmenti EP, et al. Bladder versus enteric drainage of exocrine secretions in pancreas transplantation: a retrospective analysis of the united network for organ sharing database. Pancreas. 2018;47(5):625–30.

49. Smets YF, Westendorp RG, van der Pijl JW, de Charro FT, Ringers J, de Fijter JW, et al. Effect of simultaneous pancreas-kidney transplantation on mortality of patients with type-1 diabetes mellitus and end-stage renal failure. Lancet Lond Engl. 1999;353(9168):1915–9.

50. Starzl TE, Iwatsuki S, Shaw BW, Greene DA, Van Thiel DH, Nalesnik MA, et al. Pancreaticoduodenal transplantation in humans. Surg Gynecol Obstet. 1984;159(3):265–72.

51. Stratta RJ, Farney AC, Rogers J, Orlando G. Immunosuppression for pancreas transplantation with an emphasis on antibody induction strategies: review and perspective. Expert Rev Clin Immunol. 2014;10(1):117–32.

52. Sutherland DE, Gruessner RW, Dunn DL, Matas AJ, Humar A, Kandaswamy R, et al. Lessons learned from more than 1,000 pancreas transplants at a single institution. Ann Surg. 2001;233(4):463–501.

53. Sutherland DE, Sibley R, Xu XZ, Michael A, Srikanta AM, Taub F, et al. Twin-to-twin pancreas transplantation: reversal and reenactment of the pathogenesis of type I diabetes. Trans Assoc Am Phys. 1984;97:80–7.

54. Vaidya A, Muthusamy AS, Hadjianastassiou VG, Roy D, Elker DE, Moustafellos P, et al. Simultaneous pancreas--kidney transplantation: to anticoagulate or not? Is that a question? Clin Transpl. 2007;21(4):554–7.

55. White SA, Shaw JA, Sutherland DER. Pancreas transplantation. Lancet Lond Engl. 2009;373(9677):1808–17.

56. Yabe SG, Fukuda S, Takeda F, Nashiro K, Shimoda M, Okochi H. Efficient generation of functional pancreatic β-cells from human induced pluripotent stem cells. J Diabetes. 2017;9(2):168–79.

57. Zhao M, Muiesan P, Amiel SA, Srinivasan P, Asare-Anane H, Fairbanks L, et al. Human islets derived from donors after cardiac death are fully biofunctional. Am J Transplant. 2007;7(10):2318–25.

58. NHS Blood and Transplant website. www.odt.nhs.uk/statistics-and-reports/organ-specific-reports/

Chapter 4
Liver Transplantation

Rafael Díaz-Nieto and Krishna Menon

4.1   Introduction

Thomas Starzl was the first surgeon to successfully perform a liver transplantation back in 1967. Only 1 year later, Sir Roy Calne performed the first liver transplant in Europe. It took place in Cambridge in 1968. This success came after some fatal attempts in 1963 (the first one, a child with biliary atresia who died 5 h after the operation) where some surgeons described this procedure as an *"impossible operation"*. Technical improvements especially related to veno-venous bypass made the operation feasible and allowed patients to survive the operation. Subsequent developments in inmunosupression made long-term survival possible.

R. Díaz-Nieto (✉)
Hepatobiliary Surgery Unit, Aintree University Hospital, Liverpool, UK

Liver Transplant Unit Royal Free Hospital, London, UK
e-mail: rafael.diaz-nieto@nhs.net

K. Menon
Institute of Liver Studies, King's College Hospital, London, UK

© Springer Nature Switzerland AG 2019   157
R. Díaz-Nieto (ed.), *Procurement and Transplantation of Abdominal Organs in Clinical Practice*, In Clinical Practice, https://doi.org/10.1007/978-3-030-21370-1_4

4.2   Indications for Liver Transplantation

The indication for liver transplantation is loss of metabolic function and liver failure. This most commonly occurs due to chronic liver disease but it can also present as an acute event. Any disease that can potentially damage liver function irreversibly (chronic liver disease) or, despite being reversible, represents a life threatening condition (acute liver failure) would be considered an indication for liver transplantation. The one exception to the situation where transplantation can be indicated despite the preservation of liver function is the presence of liver malignancies either primary liver cancer or metastatic liver tumours.

However, not every patient with impaired liver function or liver tumours needs, or would benefit from, a liver transplant. In principle, only patients with an expected survival equal to or less than a year or when the symptoms related to the liver disease represents a significant deterioration of their quality of life will meet the indication criteria for liver transplantation. This is the concept of End Stage Liver disease and it needs to be differentiated from specific medical diagnoses.

4.2.1   Medical Diagnosis

4.2.1.1   Cirrhosis

Cirrhosis is the final histopathological diagnosis of chronic liver disease and the most common indication that leads to transplantation. It is a very complex transformation of a healthy liver into a fibrotic non-functioning liver. The normal lobular architecture of the liver is replaced by a nodular configuration due to the presence of widespread fibrotic septa. However, cirrhosis alone is not an indication for transplantation and only when there are symptoms related to the presence of portal hypertension and decompensated cirrhosis then transplantation can be considered. Typical symptoms of decompensation include encephalopathy, ascites and variceal bleeding.

Any disease that can potentially cause cirrhosis would therefore be an indication for transplantation. The most common causes of cirrhosis are:

Infectious Diseases

One of the most common cause of chronic liver disease and the main indication for transplantation worldwide. Chronic hepatitis can evolve into cirrhosis irrespective of the origin. Viral hepatitis is the most common identifiable infection and the most common viruses are hepatitis Virus C (HVC), hepatitis Virus B (HVB), hepatitis Virus A (HVA), hepatitis Virus E (HVE) and hepatitis virus D (HVD). They can present in isolation or as a concomitant infection.

Alcohol

The burden of alcohol related liver disease is increasing worldwide. There is a wide spectrum of liver injury from alcoholic hepatitis, alcoholic steato-hepatitis to alcoholic cirrhosis. Again, it can present in the chronic setting but also as an acute event.

Traditional debates around indication of alcohol related liver disease still persist. The need of a period of abstinence, the risk of lack of adherence to treatment and recidivism are still unresolved questions. Evidence however has demonstrated that transplantation for alcohol related liver disease offers a significant survival benefit and it is cost-effective.

Non-Alcoholic Steato-Hepatitis (NASH)

It is the end of the spectrum of a more benign condition called non-alcoholic fatty liver disease (NAFLD). In the absence of alcohol consumption and other risk factors like viral hepatitis, NAFLD progress to fibrosis and cirrhosis. Clearly associated with more complex metabolic disorders including obesity and diabetes, NASH is currently an increasing indication for transplantation in western countries.

Primary Sclerosing Cholangitis (PSC)

PSC is a complex disease that commonly develops a cholestatic pattern that may lead to significant fibrosis, cirrhosis and liver failure. It is of unknown aetiology and related to ulcerative colitis (UC). It carries an increased risk of primary liver malignancy and, in the presence of UC, increased risk of colorectal cancer.

Primary Biliary Cholangitis (PBC)

Previously described as primary biliary cirrhosis is an autoimmune disease that is ostly medically managed and over the years there has been a reduction in the need for transplantation. However, in the presence on unmanageable symptoms (pruritus) and end stage liver disease, transplantation is still the only curative option.

Autoimmune Hepatitis

As with PBC, medical management of autoimmune hepatitis has significantly improved. However, it remains as indication for transplantation if there is progression to decompensated liver disease.

Metabolic Disorders

- Alpha 1 antitripsin deficiency: it is one of the metabolic disorders that is an indication for liver transplantation. Although respiratory symptoms are significantly more common than liver decompensation presentation can be predominantly with end stage liver disease. In this scenario, liver transplantation alone can be indicated and it has proven to reduce the severity and progression of the respiratory symptoms. In the presence of both, liver and respiratory failure, Alpha 1 antitripsin deficiency is an indication of combined liver and lung transplantation.
- Cystic fibrosis (CF): up to 50% of patients with CF may develop a degree of liver disease, however only 5–7% will progress to cirrhosis and an even smaller percentage

will require transplantation. Depending on the extension of the disease and CF related respiratory disease; combined liver and lung transplantation is sometimes required.

- Primary hyperoxaluria type 1. A metabolic liver disorder leads to chronic kidney disease with otherwise preserved liver function. It is commonly the renal dysfunction that leads to transplantation although as the metabolic defect is in the liver a combined liver and kidney transplant is indicated. Small series suggest that combined liver and kidney transplantation offer better long-term survival, especially in the paediatric population.

- Familiar Amyloid Polyneuropathy (FAP). This is a very rare metabolic condition that allows an almost unique procedure called Domino transplant. These patients present with a progressive neuropathy related to amyloid deposits. The amyloid precursor is a mutated protein that is released from the liver (mutated transthyretin). Liver transplantation has proven to clear this protein from the circulation and therefore control the progression of the disease. The additional peculiarity is that the liver harvested from the FAP patient is otherwise healthy and can therefore be use for a different recipient. The patient with FAP would receive a cadaveric organ and the FAP liver would be transplanted into another recipient (Domino transplant).

- Others metabolic liver disorders that are indications for transplantation are: hemochromatosis, Wilson's disease, acute intermittent porphyria, Crigler-Najjar syndrome, tyrosinaemia and atypical haemolytic uremic syndrome-1.

4.2.1.2   Malignant Tumours

This would merit a chapter on its own due to the complexity and controversies around this indication. Potential risk of tumour recurrence and progression related to immunosuppression are the key aspects. Liver limited only disease is probably the only accepted situation.

- Hepatocellular Carcinoma (HCC): HCC is the most common primary liver tumour and the main indication for liver transplantation for malignancy. Different criteria and indications for transplantation are constantly being reviewed. One of the most routinely used algorithms is the Barcelona Clinic Liver Cancer staging for HCC. Additionally, there are other inclusion criteria based on outcomes after transplantation aimed at identifying those patients that will benefit most from liver transplantation. Table 4.1 summarises some of the worlwide listing criteria for HCC but the Milan Criteria form the basis for most protocols.
- Cholangiocarcinoma: is a very controversial indication for transplantation and not widely accepted in most countries. Some pioneering series from United States suggested long-term survival benefit after transplantation for unresectable hilar cholangiocarninoma. These results are however controversial and have not been widely reproduced. Currently, most European countries do not accept cholangiocarcinoma as an indication for transplantation.

TABLE 4.1 Worldwide transplant listing criteria for HCC

Transplant criteria	Milan Criteria	UNOS Modified criteria/pTNM	UCSF	Up-to-seven
Inclusion criteria	1 tumour ≤5 cm 3 tumours <3 cm No vascular invasion	T1: 1 tumour ≤1.9 cm T2: 1 tumour >2 cm and <5 cm or <3 tumours ≤3 cm	1 tumour ≤6.5 cm ≥2 tumours <4.5 cm Sum of diameters ≤8 cm	Sum of number of tumours and maximun diameter ≤7
Exclusion criteria	1 tumour >5 cm 3 tumours >3 cm Vascular invasion	T3: 1 tumour >5 cm or >1 tumour >3 cm T4a: ≥4 tumours T4b: vascular invasion	1 tumour >6.5 cm >2 tumours >4.5 cm Sum of diameters >8 cm	Sum of number of tumours and maximun diameter >7

UNOS Unitied Network for Organ Sharing, *UCSF* University California San Francisco

- Colorectal Liver metastases (CRLM): previously considered as one of the indications, rapid progression of the disease related to inmunosuppression has precluded colorectal liver metastases to be an indication for transplantation. Recent advantages in chemotherapy and understanding of tumour biology have allowed this indication to be re-explored. CRLM as an indication is currently being explored by the Scandinavian transplant network within the setting of a clinical trial.
- Metastatic neuroendocrine tumours to the Liver (NET): patients with liver limited disease may benefit from liver transplantation if the burden of the disease is limited to the liver and deemed unresectable. Some series are reporting long-term survival benefit with transplantation but with a high rate of recurrence.

4.2.1.3 Others

Any diseases that can damage the liver parenchyma irreversibly are potential indications such as:

- Polycystic liver disease: commonly associated with polycystic kidney disease. Liver magnetic resonance (MR) imaging can identify liver cysts in up to 80% of patients with polycystic kidney disease and cerebral aneurysms but it can also present as an autosomal dominant hereditary disorder only affecting the liver. Presentation is very variable and it is commonly the presence of symptoms related to a large size of the tumours the indication for treatment. If associated with polycystic kidney disease, combined liver and kidney transplant may be indicated. Liver transplant alone is indicated in symptomatic patients (early satiety, pain or debilitating mobility due the weight and size of the polycystic liver) or uncommonly hepatic synthetic dysfunction.
- Caroli's disease: this congenital sacular dilatation of the intrahepatic bile ducts can lead to recurrent cholangitis and rarely lead to cirrhosis. End stage liver disease can represent indication for transplantation with some reports that Caroli's disease in itself can be a risk factor for cholangiocarcinoma.

- Liver adenomatosis. Similarly to polycystic liver disease, hepatic adenomatosis (more than 10 hepatic adenomas) is not an indication on its own. However the normal liver parenchyma can be completely replaced by liver adenomas leading to liver failure.
- Liver giant haemangiomas. Few cases are reported in the literature where giant heamangiomas have required transplantation.
- Liver ischaemia. Better described in paediatric population, liver ischaemia can evolve to complete liver necrosis and acute liver failure. Commonly related to hypoxic/hypoperfusion events it can also be the final consequence of a hypethrombotic status.
- Budd Chiari syndrome – is a condition with occlusion of the hepatic veins that can lead to acute or chronic hepatic failure and be indication for transplantation when more conservative approaches (anticoagulation treatment or interventional procedures like porto-systemic shunts) are not feasible or unsuccessful.
- Liver Trauma. Grade V liver trauma with a complete destruction of the liver parenchyma or irreparable injury to the hepatic hilum might be an exception in liver transplantation. As described below, the patient might survive the initial presentation and after vascular control (commonly requiring porto-caval shunt) and following anaesthetic/intensive care resuscitation, transplantation can be considered.

4.2.1.4   Acute Liver Failure

Acute liver failure represents a life threatening condition. It is defined as an acute liver injury that leads to impaired synthetic function and encephalopathy in the absence of cirrhosis or chronic liver disease.

Causes of the acute liver failure are numerous (Table 4.2). However the most common aetiology for acute liver failure is drug induced liver failure. Acetaminofen-Paracetamol poisoning is the most common drug responsible for acute liver failure.

TABLE 4.2 Common causes of acute liver failure

Drug induced	Viral infections	Others
Alcohol	Hepatitis A,B,C,E	Acute fatty liver
Acetaminophen	Cytomegalovirus (CMV)	Lymphoma
Isoniazid	Epstein-Barr virus (EBV)	Ischaemic hepatitis
Propylthiouracil	Herpes virus	Acute Budd-Chiari syndrome
Phenytoin		Autoimmune liver disease
Valproate		

The clinical presentation can vary but encephalopathy is a constant feature. The clinical condition is potentially reversible, however early referral to a transplant centre is imperative as the risk of mortality is high if untreated. Initial management is medical, in a specialist intensive care unit but if there are no signs of recovery liver transplantation must be considered. King's College criteria for transplantation distinguishes Acetaminofen from non-Acetaminofen related liver failure (Table 4.3).

4.2.2   End Stage Liver Disease

This is a concept that is aimed at establishing a cut-off point to consider transplantation. Not every patient with chronic liver disease will develop cirrhosis and not every patient with cirrhosis will require a transplant. The idea of end stage liver disease represents the serious and irreversible deterioration of liver function that carries a risk of death higher than 50% within 12 months. This is commonly related to the development of complications of portal hypertension such as ascites, variceal bleeding or encephalopathy.

TABLE 4.3 Kings College Hospital criteria for transplantation for acute liver failure

Non Acetaminophen acute liver failure		Acetaminophen acute liver failure
INR >6.5 (PT >100 s)	**OR** the presence of 3 of the below factors: Age <10 or >40 >7 days of evolution INR >3.5 (PT >50s) Bilirubin >17.5 mg/dL Drug induced	Arterial pH <7.3 **OR** INR >6.5 (PT >100 s) **OR** Serum Creatinin >3.4 mg/dL with grade ¾ encephalopathy **OR** Arterial lactate >3.5 mmol/L at 4 h **OR** Arterial lactate >3 mmol/l at 12 h after fluid resuscitation.

Many models have tried to quantify this. Probably the most relevant is the Model for End Stage liver Disease (MELD), which tries to quantify the degree of liver deterioration with a mathematical model (Formula 1). Original studies demonstrated that MELD scores of 14 or below could potentially have the best survival of those patients being transplanted and therefore many countries considered this score as a baseline for transplantation.

Formula 1: MELD calculation

$$MELD = 0.957 \times Log^e\left(creatinine\,mg/dL\right)$$
$$+ 0.378 \times Log^e\left(bilirubin\,mg/dL\right)$$
$$+ 1.120 \times Log^e\left(INR\right) + 0.643$$

There are some modifications to the original MELD scores that add some other variables with the intention of predicting survival. Most common ones are UKMELD (United Kingdom adaptation including plasma sodium levels), Na-MELD and the adaptation of MELD to paediatric patients: PMELD.

4.3 Organ Allocation

4.3.1 Indications for Liver Transplantation

The basis behind including a patient on the transplant waiting list is related to likelihood of survival post-liver transplant and mortality without a liver transplant. In principle, a patient should be considered for transplantation if the expected 5 year survival with a liver transplant is >50% or the expected 1 year mortality without a transplant is >9% based on UKELD. European guidelines suggest that any liver related disease with a life expectancy less than 1 year or a significant impaired quality of life due to symptoms should be considered criteria for consideration of liver transplantation.

Acute liver failure

Acute liver failure is a life-threatening condition and in most cases liver transplantation is the only curative option. All the transplant networks include a protocol and system of allocation of organs to acute liver failure patients to benefit from a super-urgent liver transplant. Commonly based at national or international levels, the need of an organ can be considered super-urgent (potential death within 24 h without a transplant). These allocation systems need to cover a wide variety of indications from described acute liver failure related to paracetamol intoxication to acute liver failure post transplantation (primary non-function, hepatic artery thrombosis, etc). Accepting variations between countries and systems, the inclusion criteria in the United Kingdom is based on several categories (Table 4.4).

TABLE 4.4 NHSBT Criteria for transplantation for acute liver failure

Category	Diagnosis	Criteria
Category 1	Paracetamol overdose	pH <7.25 more than 24 h after overdose and after fluid resuscitation
Category 2	Paracetamol overdose	Co-existing prothrombin time >100 s or INR >6.5, and serum creatinine >300 μmol/l or anuria, and grade 3–4 encephalopathy
Category 3	Paracetamol overdose	Significant liver injury and coagulopathy following exclusion of other causes of hyperlactatemia (e.g. pancreatitis, intestinal ischemia) after adequate fluid resuscitation: arterial lactate >5 mmol/l on admission and >4 mmol/l 24 h later in the presence of clinical hepatic encephalopathy.
Category 4	Paracetamol overdose	Two of the three criteria from category 2 with clinical evidence of deterioration (e.g. increased ICP, FiO2 >50%, increasing inotrope requirements) in the absence of clinical sepsis
Category 5	Favourable non-paracetamol aetiologies such as acute viral hepatitis or ecstasy/cocaine induced ALF	Presence of clinical hepatic encephalopathy is mandatory and: prothrombin time >100 s, or INR >6.5, or any three from the following: age >40 or <10 years; prothrombin time >50 s or INR >3.5; any grade of hepatic encephalopathy with jaundice to encephalopathy time >7 days; serum bilirubin >300 μmol/l.

TABLE 4.4 (continued)

Category	Diagnosis	Criteria
Category 6	Unfavourable non-paracetamol aetiologies such as sero-negative or idiosyncratic drug reactions	(a) prothrombin time >100 s, or INR >6.5, or (b) in the absence of clinical hepatic encephalopathy then INR >2 after vitamin K repletion is mandatory and any two from the following: age >40 or <10 years; prothrombin time >50 s or INR >3.5; if hepatic encephalopathy is present then jaundice to encephalopathy time >7 days; serum bilirubin >300 μmol/l.
Category 7	Acute presentation of Wilson's disease, or Budd-Chiari syndrome	A combination of coagulopathy, and any grade of encephalopathy
Category 8	Hepatic artery thrombosis on days 0–21 after liver transplantation	
Category 9	Early graft dysfunction on days 0–7 after liver transplantation	AST >10,000, INR >3.0, arterial lactate >3 mmol/l, absence of bile production
Category 10	The total absence of liver function (e.g. after total hepatectomy)	

(continued)

TABLE 4.4 (continued)

Category	Diagnosis	Criteria
Category 11	Any patient who has been a live liver donor (NHS entitled) who develops severe liver failure within 4 weeks of the donor operation	

4.3.2   Contra-Indications for Liver Transplantation

Absolute contraindications for liver transplantation are: significant cardiopulmonary disease that would preclude patients from surgery; presence of widespread malignancy or previous malignancies with no potential for cure; and severe active sepsis. Age, human immunodeficiency virus (HIV) infection (HIV can be an indication as well so we need to be clear re active HIV versus treated HIV with liver disease) and extreme body mass index (BMI) are relative contraindications and should be assessed individually depending on the expertise of the centre.

Active substance abuse (such as cannabis, heroin) is a contraindication for transplantation. Detailed assessment by a specialist team is required to assess this condition as active substance abuse might compromise future graft function and adherence to treatment. Ex-drug abusers can be considered eligible for transplantation if a period of abstinence (usually at least 6 months) combined with a favourable psycho-social assessment is demonstrated. Recognized replacement therapies such as methadone maintenance may be acceptable in individual cases after discussion at multidisciplinary team meetings (MDT).

Alcohol abuse as an indication for liver transplant has often been debated. Alcohol abuse can be the primary cause of end stage liver disease or may have a co-factor such Non-Alcoholic Steatohepatitis (NASH) or hepatitis C. The current UK policy is that candidates with alcohol related liver disease would need to demonstrate a minimum period of abstinence for at least 6 months. Evidence suggests that shorter periods of abstinence, family background of alcoholism and lack of social network are factors that would increase the risk of relapse.

Liver transplantation for acute liver failure due to acute alcoholic hepatitis has been considered controversial as there is no period of abstinence and there could be a higher risk of recidivism. However, attempts to set up and use protocols in the UK to offer liver transplant in this scenario have not been successful.

Other potential contraindications that merit discussions via the MDT include lack of social support, high risk behaviour, and significant porto-mesenteric thrombosis with no reconstructive options or extremely advanced disease (MELD >30).

4.3.3 Systems for Organ Allocation

Probably one of the challenges for the liver transplant surgeon is the decision making process around accepting or declining an organ for transplantation and matching the organ to the best possible recipient. Recipient inclusion into a waiting list is commonly based on a multidisciplinary approach where every patient is assessed individually with regards to the listing criteria, a full anaesthetic assessment and type of grafts that would be suitable.

At the very beginning of liver transplant programmes, time on the waiting list was probably the main consideration to prioritise recipients. This disadvantaged patients with more advanced disease and mortality on the waiting list became a significant issue. That situation evolved to recipient-based allocation systems (like the current MELD system) where the severity of the disease would be the main score over the time in the waiting list. This system also allowed the sickest patients to be prioritized and also, by the establishment of a minimal value to be listed, promoted a significant reduction of patients that were listed early. A counter argument was that this model significantly did not favour patients with better-preserved liver function but with life threatening condition such as HCC or poor quality of life related to symptoms. These indications were then considered exceptions and additional points were given so they could be prioritised on the list. Nowadays, more precise knowledge of donor and recipient risk factors add a lot of variables that will impact on the final outcome and the transplant community understand that recipient-based allocations systems are not ideal. Unfortunately, the perfect donor-recipient matching system is yet to be defined and every country or region has its own adaptation of these models.

The current allocation system that has been introduced in the UK since April 2018 uses the 'Transplant Benefit Score (TBS)' that matches a available organ nationally with a recipient who would benefit the most based on the scores. The system is under audit and early results show that there has been a significant reduction in mortality on the waiting list although this is still to be time tested. Patients within the superurgent category of listing would be listed and treated as before with no changes to the policy.

Different rules and policies among countries need consideration. Patients-based models like UNOS (United Network for Organ sharing) differ from Centres-based (or zonal-based) models like most of the regions in Europe (Scanditransplant, Eurotransplant or Spain (ONT)). They all include a national-regional escalation for medical emergencies (acute liver failure) and a degree of priority over the donors within the centre's region.

4.3.4   Living Donor Specific Criteria

Selection of adequate donors is crucial for transplantation. All the efforts of the process rely on the safety of the donor and their future health is the main aim of this type of transplantation.

Living donors must be healthy people whom a liver resection will not threaten their health and who could safely tolerate a liver resection without ameliorating their quality of life.

There are separate donor and recipient advocating teams for assessment. The donor assessment is coordinated by the living donor co-ordinator (LDC) who is the initial point of contact for potential donors and recipients requiring information. The LDC provides information on donation, evaluation, risks, outcome and ensures the donor enquiry is voluntary and without promise of reward.

4.4   Preoperative Work-up For Recipients

In parallel to the investigations related to the indication for transplantation, a more detail assessment takes place to elucidate if a patient is fit for the intervention. Many aspects needs to be considered including nutritional status, social support, specific anatomical variations among others and all them need to be discussed at MDT. Table 4.5 summarizes some of the most important test and assessment but some transplant units may have slightly small variations in their protocols. Once a patient is listed and is active in the waiting list, it is compulsory to start routine clinic reviews and update some of these investigations (specially blood tests related to MELD score) and act accordingly (modify patient's priority in the list).

Special consideration requires the use of HBV immunization for recipients who have not previously received vaccination. Immune status should be assess in every patient but in the event of a HBV mismatch between donor and recipient at the time of transplantation Hepatitis B immunoglobulin (HBIg) is required as prophylaxis during the procedure and the immediate postoperative period. The protocol includes a first dose of 4.000 units of HBIg given intravenously at the an-hepatic phase (period when the recipient's liver has been

TABLE 4.5 Summary of basic and specific preoperative tests and assessments of recipients

Laboratory tests	Specific tests	Special assessments
Full blood count	Chest X-Ray and ECG	Anaesthetic opinion (fitness for surgery)
Liver function tests	Echocardiogram	Social services (social support)
Renal function	CPET	Alcohol services
Biochemistry (including glucose)	CT angiogram (for diagnosis of malignancies and evaluation of anatomy)	Psychiatry
Clotting screen	MR/MRCP (complimentary to CT if required by surgeon)	Nutritionists and Dietician
Virology and immunizatiomn status (HVC,HVB,HIV,EBV,CMV,etc)	EEG	
Blood gases	Pulmonary function	
Tumour markers	Colonoscopy (if PSC)	
Blood group and HLA type	Bacterial screen (cultures if sepsis)	
Bone prophile (including vitamin D)		

VHC hepatitis virus C, *HVB* hepatitis virus B, *HIV* human immunodeficiency virus, *EBV* Epstein Barr virus, *CMV* Citomegalovirus, *ECG* electrocardiogram, *CPET* cardiopulmonary exercise test, *CT* computed tomography, *MR/MRCP* magnetic resonance/cholangiopancreatography, *PSC* primary sclerosing cholangitis removed and the donor's liver has not been implanted), a second dose immediately after the operation and then once daily to complete 8 doses.

Finally, despite potential variations between centres and countries, the process of consent is essential at this stage. The patient needs to take an informed decision whether to proceed with a liver transplantation. The patient needs to understand the basic steps of the operation and also the risk attached to the same. Nowadays, we understand that the patient needs to be made aware of the different types of donors (including those with viral infections or partial grafts) and specifically agrees to proceed with some or all of them. In this scenario the process of an informed consent can be very difficult and lengthily. Therefore, it is probably not adequate to do it on the day of surgery when a patient has been phoned and asked to come to the hospital because there is a potential organ. We strongly suggest that the patient gives consent during the preoperative period and consent is confirmed prior to proceed.

4.5   Surgical Procedure

4.5.1   Implantation

Implantation strictly refers to the fact of placing the new liver in position. However being liver transplantation an orthotopic transplant, it requires extraction of the diseased liver prior to the implantation of the donor liver. There is one exception to this rule, the auxiliary transplant. In this case, two-thirds of the native liver is removed, the remnant native liver remains in place and the liver from the donor is placed adjacent to it.

4.5.1.1   Standard Liver Transplantation

Initial hepatectomy is probably one of the most challenging operations of the abdominal cavity. Presence of cirrhosis, portal hypertension and vascular abnormalities makes this initial step a real challenge.

The way the hepatectomy is performed is crucial for the future implantation. Technical details of the hepatectomy differ between centres. However, to simplify them, we differentiate two main types of transplants: caval replacement technique and cava preserving technique (also known as Piggy back technique). With the first technique, the recipient hepatectomy is performed including the suprarenal portion of the cava up to the insertion of the hepatic veins. This will obviously require the donor cava to be anastomosed in an anatomical manner to the recipient cava (Fig. 4.1). Traditionally, this procedure had to be performed under complete vascular exclusion of the liver and the patient was placed on veno-veno bypass. Evolution of anaesthesia and surgical outcomes in liver transplantation allowed this procedure to be performed without the need of bypass but with a period of full occlusion of the recipient's cava.

Alternatively, with the Piggy back technique, the recipient's cava will be preserved and the donor's cava would be anastomosed to the anterior face of the recipient's cava (details below). This approach requires a more meticulous

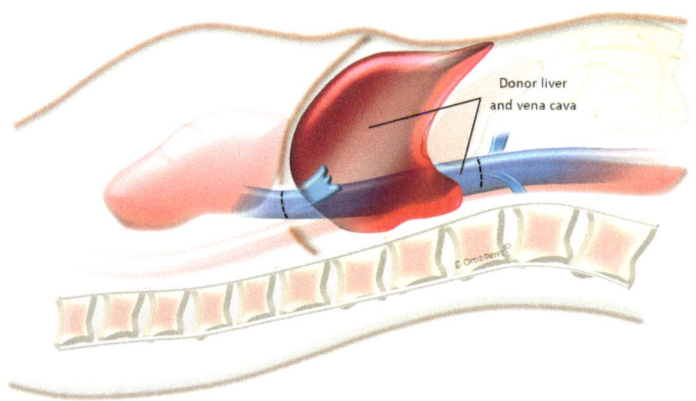

FIGURE 4.1 Illustration of classical implantation with cava replacement

mobilization of the liver from the entire length of the supra-renal cava. Clamping can then take place at the level of the hepatic veins allowing preservation of caval flow. The advantage of this technique is haemodynamic stability and potential renal function protection.

Irrespective of the chosen technique, the aim of the hepatectomy is to remove the diseased liver, preserving and identifying the vascular structures that need to be anastomosed to the donor's liver, namely: portal vein (PV), hepatic artery (HA), bile duct and hepatic veins. There may be variations between centres but it always includes full mobilization of the liver and division of all the ligaments (round, falciform, coronary and triangular ligaments), dissection of the porta hepatis and division of the portal vein, hepatic artery and bile duct plus or minus resection/dissection of the hepatic veins or cava vein. The degree of hilar dissection is also debatable with low levels of evidence underpinning it. Some centres preclude a cross clamp and division of the full hilum with no dissection at this point. This would facilitate a faster hepatectomy but will require the identification and dissection of the inflow structures at a later stage (commonly during the anhepatic phase). Some centres would prefer a full dissection of the hilum and identification of all the structures before division. This allows the dissection to be performed while the inflow is preserved, theoretically reducing the anhepatic phase. A common aspect of both techniques is that division of the inflow structures is performed as proximal to the liver as possible. Preservation of a good length of blood vessels can be crucial for the future implantation as sometimes there may be a shorter portal vein than expected (commonly in combined liver and pancreas retrieval), vascular anatomical variations or size discrepancies.

The hepatectomy finishes once the inflow and outflow are divided. A vascular clamp or equivalent at the level of hepatic veins or the suprahepatic inferior vein cava and suprarenal cava if cava is being replaced.

There is an additional surgical technique that can be very relevant and helpful during the hepatectomy: **the porto-caval**

shunt. This consists of a temporary vascular anastomosis at the time of the hepatectomy between the portal vein and the cava during the hepatectomy. This preserves the portal circulation, so reducing the portal hypertension and congestion of the bowel. Some authors also believe that this approach facilitates the mobilisation of the liver from the cava, so reducing the graft ischemic times and there evidence suggesting improved graft function with this approach. This technique is also of key importance when there is absence of collateral circulation due to lack of portal hypertension as in acute liver failure or primary non-function where the patient is critically ill and his life is threatened but a new liver is not available for transplant. In these circumstances, where the transplant team (including hepatologists, intensivists, anaesthesiologists and surgeons) understands that that the diseased liver is threatening the patient's life, there is need to proceed with the hepatectomy and wait for a donor liver. In this case the patient will stay in a prolonged anhepatic phase which can only be maintained with the presence of a porto-caval shunt. In our experience, in these cases the patients experience a relative improvement from the haemodynamic and metabolic point of view once the liver is removed and can be safely maintained with intensive care support for 24–48 h. The technique is also useful in cases of severe portal hypertension to reduce bleeding although this could be debated.

Implantation itself can then take place. However, there is a step of key importance in the process of the transplantation: **bench work (or back table work).** It is the responsibility of the transplant surgeon to check the retrieved graft and prepare it for successful implantation. This includes assessment of the organ quality, adequate perfusion, anatomical variations and potential lesions that can represent a hazard for the recipient. Typical steps required include removal of peritoneal and diaphragmatic attachments, suture of caval branches and dissection of the hilar structures to identify anatomical variations and prepare them for the implantation. If there are concerns regarding the quality of organ perfusion, then further preservation solution can be flushed via the portal vein and artery. Finally, depending on the preservation solution used (potassium rich solutions), an iso-osmotic solution should be used to flush the liver aiming to reduce the impact of these solutions at the time of reperfusion. Some centres promote the use of blood for this final flush. This procedure must always take place within the cold ischaemic phase, therefore it is compulsory that the liver is always submerged in cold preservation solution surrounded by ice. If the bench work is completed before the recipient is ready and the hepatectomy completed, the liver must be repacked and stored in ice to avoid warming.

Lastly, once the recipient liver has been removed the donor's liver is ready to be implanted., Implantation is done by anastomosing the clamped structures to the new liver. If the recipient's cava is being replaced this is the first anastomoses. Non-absorbable, continuous sutures are advised (3/0 monofilament polypropylene). In the case of caval preservation (piggy back) techniques there are more alternatives in terms of anastomosis. The initial technique was described as an end to end anastomosis from the donor's hepatic veins joining the ostium to the recipient's hepatic veins stumps. However this technique reported cases of outflow occlusion and so evolved to a side to side caval anastomosis with or without involvement of the hepatic veins stump (Fig. 4.2). There is no strong evidence comparing these techniques and they are all acceptable as they allow adequate venous drainage. Special attention requires the position of the graft at the time of the anastomosis in comparison with the "final" position of the liver. The anastomosis should facilitate adequate flow through the graft in its final position. Small rotations of the liver around the cava can easily compromise the blood flow through this type of anastomosis.

At this point some centres prefer to flush the liver again with an isotonic solution via the portal vein. This is of extreme importance if the graft has not been flushed during the bench work. Again some groups support this flush to be performed with blood rather than solutions.

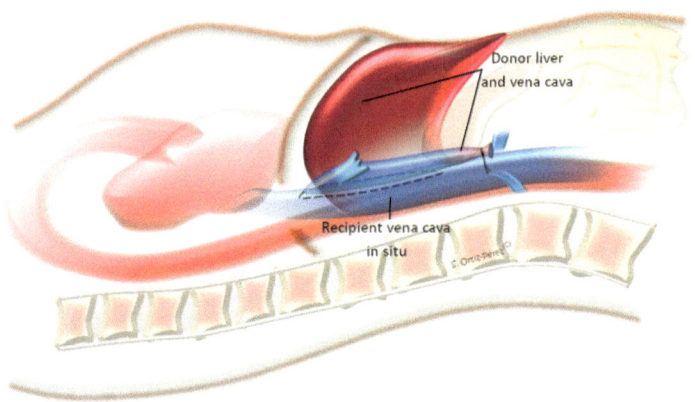

FIGURE 4.2 Illustration of "Piggy-back" technique with preservation of the recipient's cava and side to side anastomosis to the donor's cava

Attention is then turned towards the inflow. Portal vein, hepatic artery and bile duct need to be anastomosed. It is generally agreed that the bile duct are anastomosed at the end. The aim at this point is to reduce the warm ischaemia time as much as possible and therefore priority is given to the vascular structures. There are however strong controversies over whether to reperfuse the portal vein or the artery first. Most of the centres promote the early (and commonly faster) reconstruction of the portal vein allowing the liver to be reperfused immediately thereafter. The portal vein is commonly sutured in an end to end fashion (in our experience with a 5/0 or 6/0 non-absorbable polypropylene monofilament). *"Growth factor"** is strongly advised to allow for expansion of the anastomosis.

Growth factor is a known vascular technique used for venous sutures and small vessels. It can be performed either by not tying the knots or leaving them loose until the flow is reinstated in the vessel. It allows the suture line or anastomosis to expand to the right calibre of the vessel and flow. In the case of the portal vein anastomosis this can be achieved by placing a clamp above the anastomosis in the donor's portal vein and releasing the clamp in the recipient's PV.

Once venous anastomoses are secure then reperfusion can take place. After that, the caval clamps are removed first, so allowing retrograde flow through the hepatic veins. Hemodynamic stability needs to be checked at this point with the anaesthesia team and in case of haemodynamic instability the clamp should be repositioned. Adequate haemostasis of the caval anastomosis should be achieved prior to reperfusion. If the patient is stable and there is no significant bleeding, the portal vein clamp can then be removed. Hemodynamic stability needs to be re-checked as there is risk of reperfusion syndrome. Release of the portal clamp can be performed progressively allowing a smoother reperfusion ("graduated portal perfusion").

Alternative to this approach is the "artery first" reperfusion model. This is supported by some centres based on the outcome from trials that demonstrated reduced complications with this reperfusion model. There is a physiological explanation to the potential reduction of the ischaemic cholangiopathy and probably this may justify its routine use, especially for transplant from donors after circulatory death. The so-called "hepatic arterial buffer" may play a significant role on this. This mechanism of the liver microcirculation has a significant impact on vasodilatation and vasoconstriction of the portal inflow is also of great importance, even in the traditional reperfusion model when the portal vein is unclamped first. It may happen that despite appropriate outflow (good quality and calibre of the anastomosis and caval flow) the liver gets congested after portal vein reperfusion. Early arterial reperfusion may reduce this congestion.

Many techniques have been described for arterial anastomosis and basic principles of vascular surgery apply. Meticulous dissection of the vessels and attention to avoid damages or dissection of the intima are essential. Again, there is no general consensus and there may be centre variations. Continuous versus interrupted stitches are routinely used among transplant surgeons without strong evidence supporting one against the other. A classical vascular technique on which most centres base their practice is the Carrel's patch. In our centre, and in most of the groups we know, use variations of this technique to perform safe anastomoses. Elaboration of a Carrel's patch using an arterial bifurcation is commonly our standard approach. Considering a normal anatomy, places where this patch can be created are the hepatic artery bifurcation, the origin of the gastro-duodenal artery or splenic artery. The decision on where to place this anastomosis has to be made individually, aiming at an adequate size matching and flow.

Special vascular circumstances

- Arterial anatomical variations. As previously discussed in this book a large proportion of donors and recipients will present with a variant of their arterial anatomy that will require special consideration at the time of the reconstruction. Variants of the venous anatomy are possible but are significantly less frequent. Accessory left or right hepatic arteries are the most common arterial variants. This condition may simply need a more proximal anastomosis at the coeliac trunk. These types of variations are less relevant in the recipient and we only need to determine the most adequate length of the artery to create the anastomosis. In the relatively common situation where the donor has an accessory or replaced right hepatic artery that needs to be divided to allow the retrieval of the pancreas,the retrieval surgeon should make the liver transplant surgeon aware of the situation. The first option for reconstruction of this artery is an anastomosis between the accessory/replaced right hepatic artery to the gastro-duodenal artery. Therefore, both arteries have to be divided at the time of the retrieval with enough length to allow the reconstruction.

- Inadequate recipient's hepatic artery. This situation can relate to the complete occlusion or thrombosis/dissection of the artery and other situations when the recipient's hepatic artery cannot be used. In our experience the best technique to deal with this problem is the creation of an "aortic conduit" using the retrieved iliac arteries of the donor is the preferred option. These grafts are anasto-

mosed directly to the aorta (either supra-coeliac or infrar-
renal aorta) and then anastomosed to the donor's hepatic
artery.
- Recipient portal vein thrombosis. This is a relatively common situation where due to the cirrhosis or other factors
the recipient's portal vein is occluded with thrombus. The
experience of the surgical team is essential in this scenario,
as this can also be considered a relative contraindication to
transplantation in some circumstances or an indication on
its own of a multivisceral transplantation. Once in theatre,
if the calibre and walls of the vein are appropriate for an
anastomosis, the initial technique commonly used is a
thrombectomy. Again, this assessment need to be individu-
alized and every case managed differently depending on
the circumstances. Alternatives to this, when thrombectomy is not possible or the portal vein is absent, are portal
vein to varix anastomosis, arterialisation of the portal vein,
reno-portal anastomosis or a porto-caval transposition. In
the first case the portal vein is anastomosed to a dominant
varix of the patient. Secondly, the portal vein can be anastomosed to an arterial branch to warrant portal flow.
Finally the porto-caval transposition will allow caval flow
to perfuse the liver through the portal vein.

Biliary reconstruction

After the full reperfusion of the liver the only remaining
anastomosis is the biliary one. Again, there are a different
variations and possibilities when performing the biliary reconstruction. Early eras of transplantation described the use of
the gallbladder for this type of reconstruction. However, currently biliary anastomoses are routinely performed directly
with the donor's bile duct and cholecystectomy is performed
routinely, either during the bench work of after reperfusion.
Choledocho-choledochal anastomosis is the most commonly
used method, but again different variations of technique are
appropriate. From an end to end anastomosis to a side to side
anastomosis to a bilio-enteric derivation needs to be consider

and adjusted individually. Size discrepancy is the most common reason to consider these options, however some pathologies such as biliary atresia in children would obviously force the surgeon to perform a bilio-enteric anastomosis. In our experience recipients with primary sclerosis cholangitis would undergo a bilio-enteric anastomosis. However there are some series reporting that choledo-choledocal anastomosis might be safe even in this scenario. Technically anastomosis is done using a continuous or interrupted sutures. We do not recommend theuse of a "T tube" drain (Kehr drain) placed intraluminally. Some trials have suggested that the use of stents or T-Tubes drains may increase the risk of complications such as biliary stenosis. Our experience suggests that techniques should be adjusted individually to every patient and assessment of the length of the bile duct, wall thickening and diameter of the anastomosis should guide our decision on the technique.

Finally, once all the anastomoses have been performed and the liver is perfused it is essential to check on haemostais and adequate liver perfusion. Intraoperative Doppler ultrasound can be very helpful at this stage. Special consideration requires the adequate positioning of the liver. There are situations where there is a significant difference in size between the recipient's and donor's livers. In case of smaller livers we may need to consider fixation of the liver as it can be displaced producing unwanted torsions of the blood vessels (either inflow or outflow) and compromise the viability of the graft. Alternatives of this scenario are the reconstruction of the falciform ligament or the plication of the diaphragm. In case of larger size of the implanted liver it is crucial to check that the closure of the abdominal wall does not cause venous outflow or inflow issues. Too much pressure can cause a compartmental syndrome that can compromise the graft and patient survival. Consideration of a mesh repair to close the abdomen is an option. Leaving the abdomen open can be considered if the increased pressure in the abdomen is thought to be reversible (increased oedema, distended bowel). Once the new liver starts working and this situation is reversed, a primary closure can be performed safely.

4.5.1.2   Surgical Technique for Re-do Transplantation

The need of a second transplantation is relatively common. There are two different scenarios: early re-transplantation or late re-transplantation. Indications for an early re-transplantation are those related to the failure of the graft in the postoperative period. Primary non-function and hepatic artery thrombosis are the most commonest indications. Late re-transplantation relates to a chronic failure of the graft and the most common reasons are chronic rejection or recurrence of the disease.

From the technical point of view there are no variations in the technique or approach. However there are some important considerations. Commonly the hepatectomy in the case of early re-transplantation is relatively straightforward, as all the structures are already dissected. On the contrary, the hepatectomy for a late re-transplantation can be extremely challenging due to dense fibrosis obliterating the operative field. The most important technical challenge and consideration is to dissect the portal vein with great care as it any tear or damage can result in having to resort to a conduit from the superior mesenteric vein that adds signifcnt complexity to the transplant. Reconstruction in both cases can be very similar to a primary transplant or may require advanced alternatives, as described above with arterial conduits or bilio-enteric anastomoses.

4.5.1.3   Split Transplantation

The shortage of organs and the increasing waiting list for liver transplantation put a lot of pressure on the transplant community. The sharing of one organ between two recipients was a pioneering alternative a few decades ago. Initially considered as an option for paediatric recipient, this technique has now expanded and can be safely used in adults as well in graft retrieved from Donors after Brain Death (DBD).

Split transplantation is however a more complex process than a simple division of the liver for two different patients.

This should be developed by very experienced transplant units that can coordinate adult and paediatric transplantation, and the initial selection of candidates for transplantation can assess suitability for a split graft and have all their recipients matched with blood groups and weights. Additionally, the national or international protocols must include criteria that can identify the adequate donors for this approach. This is very complex and can vary among protocols. Traditional UNOS protocol considered only candidates for split:

- Donor is less than 40 years old;
- Donor is on a single vasopressor or less;
- Donor transaminases are no greater than three times the normal level
- Donor body mass index (BMI) is 28 or less.

Once the patients (recipients) and donor are correctly identified, the split of the organ can take place in two different ways: *in situ* split –before the liver has been retrieved and as part of the retrieval- or *ex situ* split –once the liver has been retrieved and the liver is split as part of the bench work-. Both techniques can be complex and risky, an adequate inflow and outflow must be guaranteed in both grafts with sufficient liver volumes. *In situ split* is basically very similar to a hepatectomy on the donor (technique can vary and depend on the surgeon's preferences) whilst the *ex situ* technique is a division of the graft through the anatomical planes. Most commonly and depending on the assessment of the liver volumes, the splits routinely performed are the division of segments 2 and 3 of the liver (for paediatric or very small adult recipients) from the rest of the liver, and secondly the split of the right and left hemilivers (segments 1 to 4 separated from segments 5 to 8).

Implantation of these grafts is essentially a full graft implantation, but with the implications of the modified anatomy. The hepatic vein stumps is anastomosed directly to the cava in most cases but again this needs to be assessed on an individual basis.

4.5.1.4   Auxiliary Liver Transplant

In patients with acute liver failure or sub-acute liver failure the concept of a hemi-hepatectomy or extended right hepatectomy to reduce toxic liver injury with liver replacement using a whole or reduced liver graft (segments 5, 6, 7, 8, 4) is a novel approach that allows for weaning of immunosuppression in the long term allowing for the native liver to regenerate. The indications are usually for paracetamol induced liver failure, acute hepatitis B or other drug induced liver injury. The patients are usually weaned off immunosuppression after the first year to 18 months and liver regeneration is monitored using CT scans and functional imaging to look for proportionate excretion is done using a HIDA scan.

4.5.2   Living Donor Liver Transplantation

Living donor liver transplantation is a relatively new approach, where the donor is a living person. The risks to the donor are an addition in this scenario and all efforts should always be made for the safety of the donor as a priority. The aim is therefore mortality/morbidity to be low for the donor. The quoted mortality for the donor undergoing a right lobe hepatectomy in living donor transplantation is 1:300 to 1:500. Although no surgical procedure is without risk, all efforts should be put in order to protect the donor.

Selection of the donor is probably the most essential part of this process. Once the donor has been identified, there is then the process of selecting the type of liver resection required. Liver volume is commonly the key aspect of this selection and is usually calculated using the MEVIS software. Traditionally used when transplanting from adults to children, volumes have not been relevant and a planned liver resection including segments II and III of the liver would be enough. Challenges are more in the adult to adult liver transplantation that carries the risk of mortality and morbidity.

The selection of the donor for living donor liver transplantation is based on the age of the donor (ideally age <50 years), general fitness (minimal or no co-morbidity), absence of steatosis in the liver and no anatomical contraindications. There may be variations of the arterial, portal and biliary anatomy that may add to the complexity of the transplant but usually these are taken into account with the overall suitability of the donor and recipient factors that may add to the risks.

Donors who are unsuitable because of an increased Body Mass Index (BMI) can sometimes be encouraged to lose weight and can be considered provided the target weight is achieved. Definitive assessment of steatosis in the liver can be made by a biopsy.

4.5.2.1   Surgical Technique for Organ Donation

Donation from a living donor consists of a hepatectomy, the resected liver being the future graft. Technically it does not differ much from an anatomical liver resection, however a very meticulous dissection is essential to warrant adequate inflow and outflow.

4.5.2.2   Organ Preservation in Living Donor Liver Transplantation

One of the greatest advantages of LDLT is the possibility of scheduling the procedure electively. This will definitely impact on shorter warm and cold ischaemia times. Ideally, the donor hepatectomy and recipient hepatectomy can happen simultaneously and as soon as the graft is removed from the donor the recipient should be ready for implantation.

4.6   Postoperative Management

4.6.1   Immunosuppression

Immunosuppression is essential after liver transplantation. It is important to get certain level of immunosuuppression to avoid rejection, but maintaining this level of immunosuppression low enough to avoid the complications related to it. On the daily basis, it becomes an individualised approach as every patient might be slightly different. We also observe variations between countries and centres where they can have specific protocols.

Most protocols will differentiate between "induction immunosuppression" and "maintenance immunosuppression." In the first case, we aim at loading the patient with immunosuppression, trying to avoid rejection during the early postoperative period. The second type of regimen starts later after the transplantation and represents a long-term treatment aiming at avoiding chronic rejection. Both regimens can be single agent based or a combination of different agents (dual or triple therapies).

Table 4.6 summarizes some of the most important agents used currently and most common side effects. Most of them require variable dosing and the exact dose is based on plasma levels. These levels need to be monitored and adjusted. In our experience, induction immunosuppres-

TABLE 4.6 Most commonly used inmunosupresants and side effects

Drug	Type/Action	Side effect
Methylprednisolone Prednisone Prednisolone	Corticoesteroid/ Anti-inflammatory	Delirium Hypertension Hyperlipidaemia Diabetes Osteoporosis
Tacrolimus	CNI	Nephrotoxicitiy Neurotoxicity
Cyclosporine	CNI	
Azathioprine	Anti-Metabolite	Bone narrow suppression
Mycophenolate Mofetil (MMF)	Anti-Metabolite	Bone narrow suppression Gastrointestinal symptoms

(continued)

TABLE 4.6 (continued)

Drug	Type/Action	Side effect
Sirolimus	mTOR inhibitor	Oedema Hyperlipidaemia Oral ulcers Impared wound healing
Everolimus	mTOR inhibitor	Oedema Hyperlipidaemia Oral ulcers Impaired wound healing
Basiliximab	Anti IL-2 monoclonal antibody	
Alemtuzumab	Anti T cell monoclonal antibody	Rapid recurrence of HVC
Anti-Thymoglobuline (ATG)	Anti T cell polyclonal antibody	Cytokine release syndrome Anaphylaxis Potential increased risk of PTLD

mTOR inhibitor mammalian target of rapamycin inhibitors, *CNI* calcineurin inhibitors

sion is based on a dual therapy of steroids and Calcineurin Inhibitors (CNI) and maintenance therapy is ideally with single drugs. Circumstances like renal failure/chronic kidney disease, nephrotoxicity of neurotoxicity might preclude a patient from CNIs and alternative treatment with Mycophenolate mofetil (MMF) or Azathioprine needs to be considered. Individual indications like autoimmune hepatitis, PSC and PBC may include low dose steroids for the long term to prevent not only rejection but recurrence. All these alternatives need to be well documented in internal or national protocols.

4.6.2 Postoperative Complications

The postoperative course of a liver transplantation is a relatively complex journey that requires a true multidisciplinary approach. In addition to the postoperative care of any surgical patient, it requires specific care and medication to monitor graft function. The addition of immunosuppression obviously impacts on the management of the patient as a whole.

Any surgical patient can have postoperative complications such as bleeding, infection and organ failure. Transplant patients also have the risk of graft failure and the specific complications of the transplant itself.

- Infectious complications: this are the most common complications in transplant patient and in many centres the most common cause of death especially in the first year post-transplantion. The immunosuppression would obviously impact on it, not only regarding the more severe infections compared to immunocompetent patients, but also the fact that there might be medical interaction between antibiotics and immunosuppressants. In this setting there is a relevant concept called the "Net State of Immunosuppression" which is the sum of congenital, acquired, metabolic, operative, and transplant-related factors for infection. Some of these factors are type, dose and duration of immunosuppression; presence of surgical devices such as drains; presence of co-infections and patient's factors that can influence the immune function.

Time of presentation is also relevant for infectious complications. Level of immunosuppression and external factors vary with time. Infectious complications during the first month are commonly associated with the surgical procedure itself. Not only the surgical site infections (wound and intra-abdominal collections), but also those related to the intervention (pneumonia, line sepsis, urinary tract infection, bacteraemia, etc.). Organisms responsible of these infections are commonly bacteria (around 50% of all cases in reported series), fungi and virus (especially *Citomegalovirus (CMV)*) that had colonized the receptor or the donor prior to the transplant. Several risk factors have been identified among published series. The most important one is the presence of a latent infection in the donor or recipient at the time of transplantation. Other relevant factors are the length of the operation, the body mass index (BMI), re-transplantation and bilio-enteric anastomosis. The period between the first month and the sixth month after transplant is time of greatest risk for opportunistic infections. Some of the most relevant ones are *Pneumocystis jirovecii,* tuberculosis, and viral infections. After 6 months, most of patient will have a more stabilized inmunosupresion levels but are still at risk of community adquired infections and also late-onset of CMV. Special relevance has at this stage the potential recurrence of viral infections such us VHC and VHB.

Another relevant aspect of the management of infectious complications in the transplanted patient is that early diagnosis is crucial. Early signs of sepsis can be non-specific and mimic other complications, such as graft failure or rejection. It is important to have a high level of awareness and a low threshold for investigation of underlying infections. The presence of previous infections in the donor and recipient implies that there is an increased incidence of multidrug resistant bacteria. Microbiological diagnosis (cultures and resistance profile) should be always pursued and early treatment is essential. Most of the transplant centres include a regimen of antibiotic prophylaxis and this should be discussed on an individual basis, but different microbiology and resistance profiles makes a unified protocol impossible.

Special mention is required with regard to postoperative CMV infection. The concept of CMV Infection (sometimes considered "reactivation" of CMV) is different from CMV disease as many patients are colonized by CMV with no evident disease. CMV disease however has significant consequences to patients that have received a liver transplant. It is associated with increased mortality in the first year postransplantation, increases the incidence of concomitant infections and promotes early recurrence of HVC. Immunity status against

CMV (CMV+ vs CMV−) is very variable among donors and recipients, therefore CMV− recipients that received a liver from a CMV+ donor, this group of patients have the highest risk of CMV infection post-transplantation. There are small variations between centres, but guidelines suggest prophylactic treatment for all high risk patients.

- Organ failure: again related to any operation, but in this case organ specific complication can be of higher incidence. For example, renal failure can be related to a increased blood loss and prolonged caval clamping, but also triggered by the use of nephrotoxic drugs like Tacrolimus.
- Hepatic artery thrombosis (HAT): this is a graft threatening complication that can quickly lead to graft failure. Reported incidences vary from 1% to 7% of transplants. The thrombosis, or the lack of flow through the hepatic artery can develop graft ischaemia and subsequent graft failure. Despite the non-surgical techniques described with the use of intra-arterial catheters for direct fibrinolysis or anticoagulation, up to 50% of patients with HAT are offered a re-intervention. Some surgeons however promote that despite best efforts to improve the recipients arterial flow (arterial grafts, re-anastomosis, etc), these techniques will not improve the flow of the graft's artery. Based on this, and sometime irrespective of these techniques, most patients would require re-listing for transplantation as a predicted graft failure/primary non-function.
- Portal vein thrombosis (PVT).

Varialble incidence of PVT is described. It also can represent a graft-threatening complication, especially in the paediatric setting. It is more common in the scenario of previously thrombosed PV or difficult anastomosis, as mentioned above, but outside the scenarios where a technical problem can be the cause of the thrombosis.

Non-occlusive thrombus may be present and indentified incidentally during a scan requested for a different reason. This thrombus however can potentially progress to a complete occlusion and unless there are clinical concerns regarding active bleeding the patient should be treated with anticoagulation.

Clinical presentations of PVT may vary from an indolent presentation with no symptoms to a rapid deterioration of the patient with evidence of graft failure. These different scenarios will guide the decision on the most adequate management. There are some series promoting conservative treatment of late presentation of the PVT in a clinically stable patient. Similarly to HAT, a complete occlusion of the portal vein with graft loss is an indication for surgical exploration aiming at a thrombectomy or refashioning of the anastomosis. Extreme cases with evident graft failure, or where there is no technical options to perform a new anastomosis would require urgent retransplantation. These last cases would probably require a multivisceral transplant.

- Primary non-Function (PNF).

Lack of synthetic function of the implanted liver is a risk in every case. In the absence of identifiable cause like HAT, PVT or rejection, the most common factors associated with PNF are prolonged ischaemia time, severe steatosis and ischaemic-reperfusion injury. It is an indication of re-transplantation in all cases as it is an unreversible condition. However, if the patient's cinical condition is such that they woukd not survive a re-transplantation then it should be avoided.

- Rejection

Improvements in immunosuppression regimens have significantly reduced the incidence of rejection, however rejection after liver transplantation from cadaveric donors still remains around 25%. This is significantly lower after living donation.

Rejection can present as super-acute, acute of chronic rejection. Super-acute rejection is commonly immediately after transplantation and it is usually the expression of a complete incompatibility. Risk factors for acute rejection include: inadequate immunosuppression, diagnosis of primary biliary cirrhosis and primary sclerosing cholangitis. The acute presentation takes place within the first postoperative days (mostly first 90 days post-transplant) and is usually diagnosed due to progressive deterioration of the liver function. The gold standard for the diagnosis is histological confirmation (via liver biopsy) and sometime it is compulsory for the differential diagnosis with primary non-function and other causes of graft failure. Initial, and commonly definitive, treatment consists of high dose intravenous steroids. Up to 90% of patients will respond to treatment (either with a single course of multiple courses of steroids) and there are controversial data regarding the consequences of rejection. Some series have reported that acute rejection does not impact on the final patient or graft survival, while others have published increased risk of chronic rejection and graft failure. Up to 10% of patients may develop steroid resistant rejection that will need modification of the immunosuppression and might lead to graft failure, requiring re-transplantation.

- Biliary complications

Complications related to the biliary system are relatively common. These include bile leak, biliary stricture and ischaemic cholangiopathy.

Bile leak is often a technical problem related to the biliary anastomosis. Irrespective of the technique of biliary reconstruction, there is a small risk of biliary leakage. Low volume bile leak (commonly defined as volume <500 mls/24 h) can sometimes be well tolerated by the patient and can be managed conservatively by endoscopic retrograde cholangiography (ERCP) and biliary stenting. The leak should resolve with a progressive decrease in the volume from the drain until complete resolution. Large volume bile leak or clinical deterioration of the patient requires intervention. Large volume bile leaks may represent ischaemia/necrosis of the bile duct and this condition will require surgical intervention and a new anastomosis. ERCP can be attempted or a percutaneous transhepatic cholangiography (PTC) to stent or place a catheter across the leak in the latter method. Outside the standard OLT, split grafts and Living Donor Liver Transplant

(LDLT) include an area of transected liver which can be an additional source of bile leaks. The same principles apply and conservative management can be offered against radiological or surgical management.

Biliary strictures can present in the early or late postoperative course. This condition applies only to the anastomosis unless there is an underlying cholangiopathy in the implanted graft. Progressive jaundice is the clinical presentation and will require intervention in almost all cases. Non-surgical management including endoscopic or percutaneous dilatation and insertion of stents can achieve very good results, even in the long term. However some case will require a new intervention and reconfiguration of the biliary anastomosis.

Ischaemic cholangiopathy

Ischaemic bile duct injuries are very serious complications that can lead to retransplantation. Traditional risk factors include AB0 incompatibility, HAT and ischaemia reperfusion injury, however more recently we have seen an increase incidence of this complication in relation with the increase of living donor liver transplantation and donation after circulatory death (DCD) where IC is described in up to 30% of cases.

4.7   Outcomes

4.7.1   Patient Survival

Data from the European Registry of liver transplantation including more than 120,000 patients transplanted between 1988 and 2015 reports 1, 3 and 5 years survival of 83%, 76% and 71% respectively. Longer term results of this population include a 10 years survival of 61% with 41% of the patients alive 20 years post-transplant. Similar data from the United States, with more than 160,000 patients transplanted since 1988, show 1 year survival greater that 85% and 5 year survival greater than 75%.

4.7.2 Graft Survival

Graft survival represents a more complex concept especially in the era of extended criteria donor. Data from the United States report graft survival in 1 and 7 years of 77% and 57% respectively, however there is significant difference between the type of grafts. Graft survival from DCD donors (71% at 1 year and 60% at 3 years) is significantly lower than survival of DBD donors (80% at 1 year and 72% at 3 years). However, a more detailed analysis considering the most significant risk factors (donor age, ischaemia times, etc.) allowed the identification of groups at risk within the DCD grafts. A more favourable group of donors (age ≤45 years, warm ischaemia time ≤15 min, and cold ischaemia time ≤10 hr) presents comparable graft survival to that for DBD donors (84.9% at 1 year, 75.2% at 3 years, and 69.4% at 5 years).

4.8 Additional Professional Skills for the Transplant Surgeon

The liver transplant surgeon is expected to be a very expert and skilled surgeon with wide knowledge of the pathology, the clinical scenario around the liver transplantation and an enormous variety of surgical skills to perform one of the most –if not the most- complex surgical procedures. However, beyond the medical and technical aspects of the operation, it is important to have a combination of qualities to succeed in the job.

Decision making: Probably one of the most difficult roles of the transplant surgeon is the acceptance or rejection of an organ and its adequate allocation to the most suitable recipient. Despite the allocations systems already discussed, in the era of extended criteria donors, the decision to decline or accept an organ is essential and will impact on the outcomes.

Teamplayer: Multidisciplinary teams are more and more relevant to liver transplantation. Considering the possibilities of working within a team, being comprehensive and collaborative is essential. At the same time, the surgeon has to be the team leader of this transplant team and therefore at the same time needs to be assertive, calm and show very good communication skills.

Ultimately the surgeon is responsible of the whole process of transplantation. The final assessment of the quality of the transplanted organ is his responsibility. The surgeon needs to be sure that data is stored and managed adequately, donor identity kept anonymous, ID checks, etc.

Teaching and training ability: New generations of surgeons need to be trained so there is adequate continuation of care. Seniority in transplantation is priceless and this needs to be transmitted to the future generations of surgeons.

Finally, within the era of evidence based medicine, it is expected that every transplant consultant be familiarized with the latest evidence around liver transplantation, indications and techniques and it is desirable that holding a higher degree demonstrates a research interest in the field aiming at continuously develop and improve outcomes.

4.9   Future Perspectives

Liver transplantation is definitely an evolving entity and it has continuously changed since its origins. It is obviously impossible to predict what the future of liver surgery will be but there are some aspects at present that will definitely change the future of transplantation.

The indication for transplantation is one of the key aspects that may change in the future. Current development of better treatment of viral hepatitis (specially HVC) may reduce significantly the incidence the number of transplant performed for this reason. On the contrary, western countries are suffering an endemic increase of NASH, which may become the main indication for liver transplantation. The future management of tumours like HCC is also an evolving process that will change the indication for transplantation in the oncological setting.

Presently is the development of machine perfusion devices. This approach is already in place aiming at improving outcomes in graft survival, but may also have an important role in "rescuing" organs that are not suitable for transplantation but that may recover after a period of *ex vivo*/*in vivo* perfusion. Organ shortage is a crucial problem nowadays and might be ameliorated by these new devices.

Very promising is also the advances achieved in liver regeneration and tissue engineering. Tissue printing and creation of artificial organs is becoming more and more a reality. There is still a long way ahead but all efforts are in place for a promising future of liver transplantation.

Bibliography

1. Starzl TE. In: Putnam CW, editor. Experience in hepatic transplantation. W. B. Saunders Co: Philadelphia; 1969.
2. Calne RY, Williams R. Liver transplantation in man. Observations on technique and organization in five cases. BMJ. 1968;4:535–50.
3. Penn I, Halgrimson CG, Starzl TE. Liver transplantation in man. Ann N Y Acad Sci. 1970;170:251–8.
4. European Association for the Study of the Liver. EASL clinical practice guidelines: liver transplantation. J Hepatol. 2016;64(2):433–85.
5. Martin P, DiMartini A, Feng S, et al. Evaluation for liver transplantation in adults: 2013 practice guideline by the American Association for the Study of Liver Diseases and the American Society of Transplantation. Hepatology. 2014;59(3):1144–65.
6. https://bts.org.uk/wp-content/uploads/2016/09/20_BTS_Liver_Non-alcoholic-1.pdf.
7. Mathurin P, Moreno C, Samuel D, et al. Early liver transplantation for severe alcoholic hepatitis. N Engl J Med. 2011;365:1790.
8. Kemmer N, Kaiser T, Zacharias V, Neff GW. Alpha-1-antitrypsin deficiency: outcomes after liver transplantation. Transplant Proc. 2008;40:1492.
9. Carey EJ, Iyer VN, Nelson DR, et al. Outcomes for recipients of liver transplantation for alpha-1-antitrypsin deficiency–related cirrhosis. Liver Transpl. 2013;19:1370.
10. Herlenius G, Wilczek HE, Larsson M, et al. Ten years of international experience with liver transplantation for familial amyloidotic polyneuropathy: results from the Familial Amyloidotic Polyneuropathy World Transplant Registry. Transplantation. 2004;77:64.

11. Yang JD, Larson JJ, Watt KD, et al. Hepatocellular carcinoma is the most common indication for liver transplantation and placement on the waitlist in the United States. Clin Gastroenterol Hepatol. 2017;15:767.
12. Ostapowicz G, Fontana RJ, Schiødt FV, et al. Results of a prospective study of acute liver failure at 17 tertiary care centers in the United States. Ann Intern Med. 2002;137:947.
13. Eghtesad B, Aucejo F. Liver transplantation for malignancies. J Gastrointest Cancer. 2014;45:353.
14. Fahrner R, Dennler SGC, Dondorf F, et al. Liver resection and transplantation in Caroli disease and syndrome. J Visc Surg. 2018;pii: S1878–7886(18):30079–1.
15. Tepetes K, Selby R, Webb M, et al. Orthotopic liver transplantation for benign hepatic neoplasms. Arch Surg. 1995;130:153.
16. Hakeem AR, Cockbain AJ, Raza SS, Pollard SG, Toogood GJ, Attia MA, Ahmad N, Hidalgo EL, Prasad KR, Menon KV. Increased morbidity in overweight and obese liver transplant recipients: a single-center experience of 1325 patients from the United Kingdom. Liver Transpl. 2013;19(5):551–62.
17. Bronsther O, Fung JJ, Izakis A, et al. Prioritization and organ distribution for liver transplantation. JAMA. 1994;271(2):140–3.
18. Zoghbi GJ, Patel AD, Ershadi RE, et al. Usefulness of preoperative stress perfusion imaging in predicting prognosis after liver transplantation. Am J Cardiol. 2003;92:1066.
19. Guckelberger O, Mutzke F, Glanemann M, et al. Validation of cardiovascular risk scores in a liver transplant population. Liver Transpl. 2006;12:394.
20. Krowka MJ, Mandell MS, Ramsay MA, et al. Hepatopulmonary syndrome and portopulmonary hypertension: a report of the multicenter liver transplant database. Liver Transpl. 2004;10:174.
21. Widmer JD, Schlegel A, Ghazaly M, et al. Piggy-back or cava replacement - which implantation technique protects liver recipients from acute kidney injury and complications? Liver Transpl. 2018;24:1746–56. https://doi.org/10.1002/lt.25334.
22. Pratschke S, Rauch A, Albertsmeier M, et al. Temporary intraoperative porto-caval shunts in piggy-back liver transplantation reduce intraoperative blood loss and improve postoperative transaminases and renal function: a meta-analysis. World J Surg. 2016;40(12):2988–98.
23. Moini M, Schilsky ML, Tichy EM. Review on immunosuppression in liver transplantation. World J Hepatol. 2015;7(10):1355–68.
24. https://unos.org/data/.

25. https://optn.transplant.hrsa.gov/data/view-data-reports/
    state-data/.
26. Lee K-W, Simpkins CE, Montgomery RA, et al. Factors affect-
    ing graft survival after liver transplantation from donation after
    cardiac death donors. Transplantation. 2006;82(12):1683–8.
27. Mateo R, Cho Y, Singh G, et al. Risk factors for graft survival
    after liver transplantation from donation after cardiac death
    donors: an analysis of OPTN/UNOS data. Am J Transplant.
    2006;6(4):791–6.
28. Menon KV, Hakeem AR, Heaton ND. Review article: liver trans-
    plantation for hepatocellular carcinoma - a critical appraisal of
    the current worldwide listing criteria. Aliment Pharmacol Ther.
    2014;40(8):893–902.
29. Nadalin S, Capobianco I, Panaro F, Di Francesco F, Troisi R,
    Sainz-Barriga M, Muiesan P, Königsrainer A, Testa G. Living
    donor liver transplantation in Europe. Hepatobiliary Surg Nutr.
    2016;5(2):159–75.
30. Ceresa CDL, Nasralla D, Jassem W. Normothermic machine
    preservation of the liver: state of the art. Curr Transplant Rep.
    2018;5:104–10.
31. Radtke A, Nadalin S, Sotiropoulos GC, Molmenti EP, Schroeder
    T, Valentin-Gamazo C, Lang H, Bockhorn M, Peitgen HO,
    Broelsch CE, Malagó M. Computer-assisted operative plan-
    ning in adult living donor liver transplantation: a new way to
    resolve the dilemma of the middle hepatic vein. World J Surg.
    2007;31(1):175–85.
32. Radtke A, Schroeder T, Molmenti EP, Sotiropoulos GC, Schenk
    A, Paul A, Frilling A, Lang H, Nadalin S, Peitgen HO, Broelsch
    CE, Malagó M. Anatomical and physiological comparison of liver
    volumes among three frequent types of parenchyma transection
    in live donor liver transplantation. Hepato-Gastroenterology.
    2005;52(62):333–8.
33. Czigany Z, Scherer MN, Pratschke J, Guba M, Nadalin S,
    Mehrabi A, Berlakovich G, Rogiers X, Pirenne J, Lerut J, Mathe
    Z, Dutkowski P, Ericzon BG, Malagó M, Heaton N, Schöning
    W, Bednarsch J, Neumann UP, Lurje G. Technical aspects of
    orthotopic liver transplantation-a survey-based study within
    the Eurotransplant, Swisstransplant, Scandiatransplant, and
    British Transplantation Society Networks. J Gastrointest Surg.
    2019;23(3):529–37.
34. Nasralla D, Coussios CC, Mergental H, Akhtar MZ, Butler AJ,
    Ceresa CDL, Chiocchia V, Dutton SJ, García-Valdecasas JC,

Heaton N, Imber C, Jassem W, Jochmans I, Karani J, Knight SR, Kocabayoglu P, Malagò M, Mirza D, Morris PJ, Pallan A, Paul A, Pavel M, Perera MTPR, Pirenne J, Ravikumar R, Russell L, Upponi S, Watson CJE, Weissenbacher A, Ploeg RJ, Friend PJ. Consortium for organ preservation in Europe. A randomized trial of normothermic preservation in liver transplantation. Nature. 2018;557(7703):50–6.

35. Lee EC, Kim SH, Park SJ. Outcomes after liver transplantation in accordance with ABO compatibility: a systematic review and meta-analysis. World J Gastroenterol. 2017;23(35):6516–33.

36. Lim KB, Schiano TD. Long-term outcome after liver transplantation. Mt Sinai J Med. 2012;79(2):169–89.

37. Charlton MR. Improving long-term outcomes after liver transplantation. Clin Liver Dis. 2014;18(3):717–30.